Unicompartmental Knee Arthroplasty

Unicompartmental Knee Arthroplasty

RICHARD D. SCOTT, MD
Professor of Orthopedic Surgery, Emeritus
Harvard Medical School
Boston, Massachusetts

VIVEK M. SHAH, MD
Assistant Professor of Orthopedic Surgery
Harvard Medical School
Boston, Massachusetts

ELSEVIER

Elsevier
1600 John F. Kennedy Blvd.
Ste 1800
Philadelphia, PA 19103-2899

UNICOMPARTMENTAL KNEE ARTHROPLASTY ISBN: 978-0-323-79010-9

Senior Content Strategist: Belinda Kuhn
Content Development Specialist: Rebecca Corradetti
Director, Content Development: Ellen Wurm-Cutter
Publishing Services Manager: Shereen Jameel
Senior Project Manager: Karthikeyan Murthy
Design Direction: Bridget Hoette

Printed in India.

Last digit is the print number: 9 8 7 6 5 4 3 2 1

To the knee arthroplasty surgeons of the past who have shown that unicompartmental arthroplasty is a viable and successful alternative to total knee arthroplasty in selected patients, and to the arthroplasty surgeons of the present and the future who will continue to utilize and perfect prosthetic components and surgical technique.

CONTENTS

PREFACE

Unicompartmental knee arthroplasty (UKA) has been evolving since its introduction over 50 years ago and has been controversial for most of that time. One of us (RDS) has been an experienced advocate of the procedure for over four decades. The other of us (VMS) is from the next generation of UKA surgeons and brings his perspective to allow this unique book to cover the past, present, and future of UKA.

-Richard D. Scott
-Vivek M. Shah

1

Historical Evolution of Unicompartmental Knee Arthroplasty

In the 1960s, the modern era of knee arthroplasty began with the introduction of the MGH mold femoral hemiarthroplasty pioneered at the Massachusetts General Hospital. At the same time, the McKeever metallic tibial hemiarthroplasty was being used at the Robert B Brigham hospital (now the Brigham and Womens Hospital) in patients with rheumatoid arthritis. With the advent of successful metal-to-plastic hip arthroplasty in the early 1970s, prosthetic designs were sought that were made of the same metal and plastic materials. Among these were modular components that would resurface each condyle separately, utilizing metal on the femoral side and plastic on the tibial side of the articulation. The polycentric knee and the Marmor knee were among these early designs.[1,2] Instrumentation for accurate prosthetic implantation was lacking and these modular components also provided no provision for resurfacing of the patellofemoral compartment. In fact, they often created an incongruent transition for the patella as it left the femoral trochlea to articulate with the femoral condyles in high flexion. Some of the earliest modular femoral and tibial components survived, however, by playing a role in unicompartmental replacement of either the medial or lateral compartment of the knee.

Despite being available and utilized for over five decades, unicompartmental knee arthroplasty (UKA) has been a controversial procedure since its introduction. Initial reports were discouraging regarding UKA in medial compartment osteoarthritis.[3,4] A few years later, more favorable results using the "Unicondylar" prosthesis were published from our instutution.[5] One hundred knees with 2- to 6-year follow-up were studied. Three repeat operations had been performed, for an incidence of revision of roughly 1% per year at this short follow-up. The average flexion was 114 degrees, significantly better than in any contemporary reports using bicompartmental arthroplasty. When the same series was followed at 5 to 9 years (mean 7 years), seven revisions had been performed for a revision rate continuing at 1% per year.[6] The total condylar tricompartmental experience at that time for the same follow-up also showed a revision rate of 1% per year.[7] Armed with this information, our local enthusiasm for unicompartmental arthroplasty began to grow. We felt that when the knee was exposed for arthroplasty and the patient fulfilled the criteria for unicompartmental replacement, it was reasonable to perform this procedure on these patients. By the early 1980s, approximately 10% of knee replacement patients at the Brigham with osteoarthritis underwent unicompartmental replacement.

Over the years, prosthetic design changes evolved as follow-up revealed that failures due to certain issues could be minimized by these modifications. For example, we began to see failures in obese patients. These were due to either tibial or femoral loosening. We saw some femoral components loosen by subsiding into the subchondral bone (Fig. 1.1). We recognized that the force across the knee in level gait is approximately three times body weight. This force is ideally distributed evenly to the medial and lateral compartment over the surface area provided by each compartment. The pounds per square inch force will increase if there are more pounds and fewer square inches covered by the prosthetic components. We thereby came to realize that the relatively small size of early UKA components made them vulnerable to loosening in heavy patients.

To address this issue, the unicondylar prosthesis used at the Brigham and Womens Hospital was redesigned to the "Brigham" unicompartmental knee in 1981 (Fig. 1.2). The femoral component was made 5 mm wider to better cap the subchondral bone and resist subsidence. The tibial component was a nonmodular, metal-backed component with a composite thickness starting at 6 mm (Fig. 1.3).

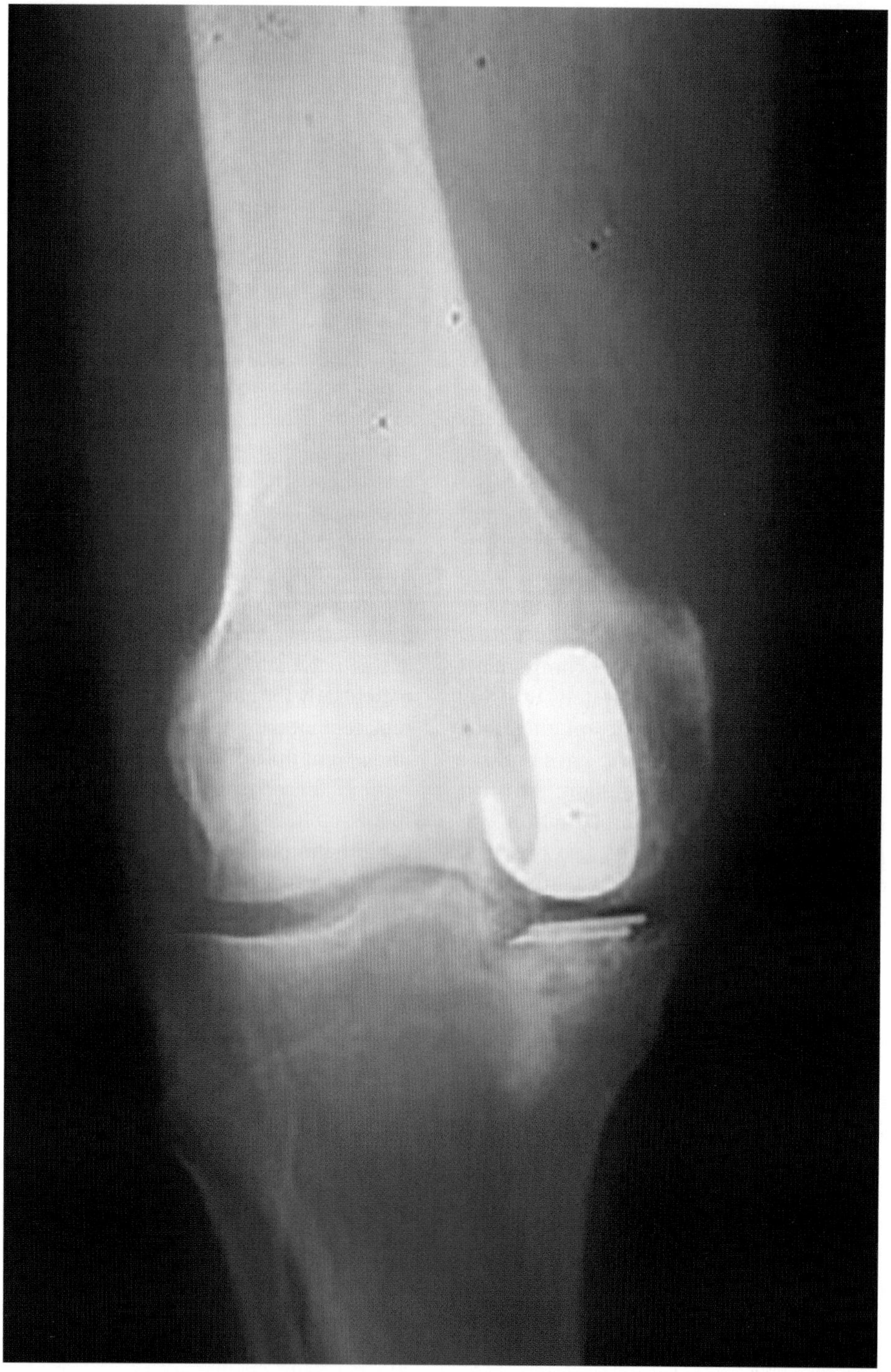

Fig. 1.1 Subsidence of the Femoral Component in a Heavy Patient. (From Scott, RD. *Total Knee Arthroplasty*. 2nd ed. Philadelphia: Saunders; 2014.)

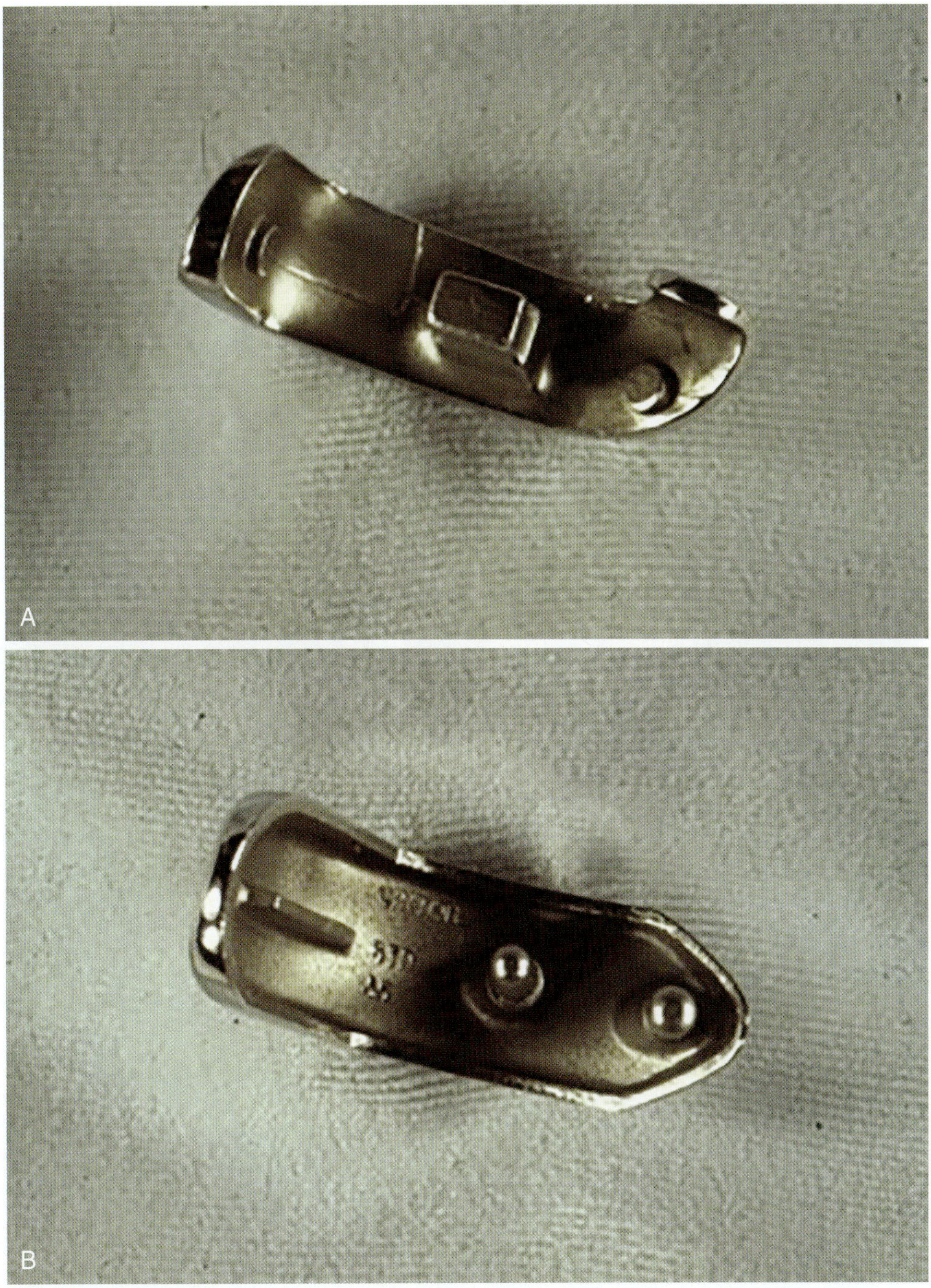

Fig. 1.2 (A) The relatively narrow runner of the unicondylar femoral component made it vulnerable to subsidence. (B) The Brigham knee was 5 mm wider to better cap the subchondral bone and resist subsidence. (From Scott, RD. *Total Knee Arthroplasty*. 2nd ed. Philadelphia: Saunders; 2014.)

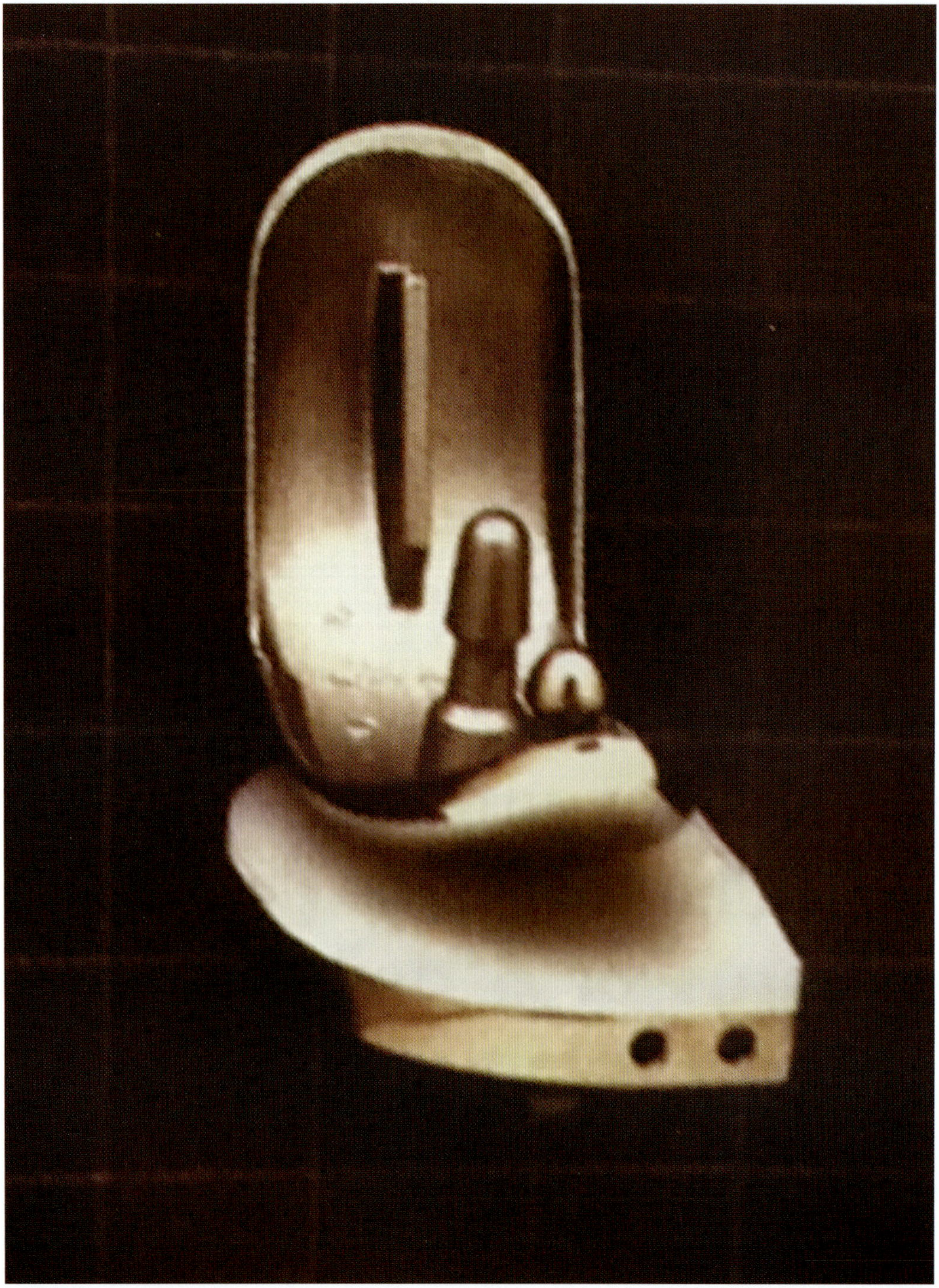

Fig. 1.3 The 6-mm metal-backed tibial component of the Brigham knee had only 2 mm of polyethylene in parts of its articulating surface.

The articulation was flat-on-flat to diminish stress on the polyethylene and increase surface contact. This prosthesis was used exclusively for the next 8 or 9 years. The specifics of its design and surgical technique taught us more important lessons about unicompartmental arthroplasty.[8]

Because the articulation was flat-on-flat, it became apparent that imprecise surgical technique was unforgiving. If the component articulating surfaces were not parallel during weight bearing, edge-loading would occur, leading to accelerated wear of the polyethylene (Fig. 1.4).

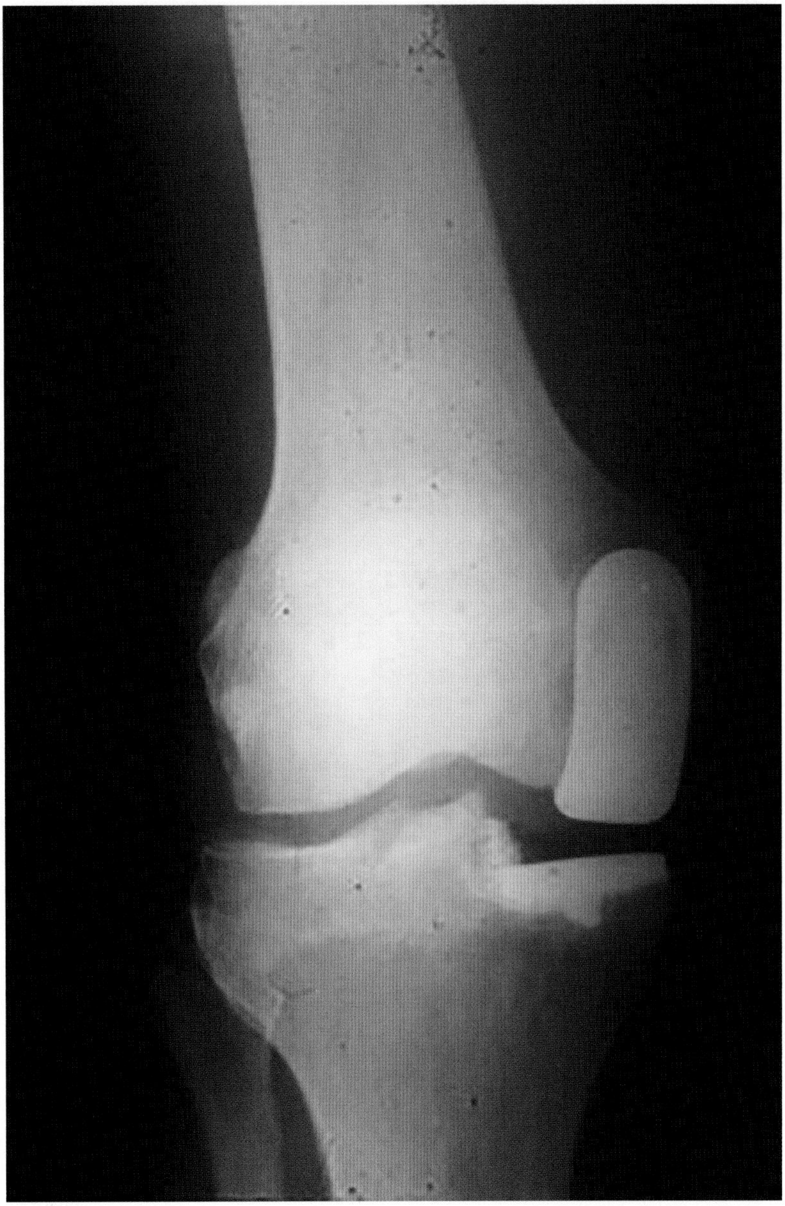

Fig. 1.4 Poor Surgical Technique Can Lead to Edge-Loading of a Flat-on-Flat Articulation.

This led to the evolution of round-on-relatively flat articulations where the kinematics of the articulation could be accommodated without edge-loading while still providing an acceptable wear surface. It also led to the development of a mobile bearing articulation in the 1980s that would provide maximum bearing contact to decrease wear potential while allowing the dissipation of torsional stresses on the polyethylene.

As the years pass, designs have continued to evolve to maximize early results and extend the longevity of the arthroplasty. Early designs usually had only two sizes, small and large. Many modern systems have as many as five sizes of both femoral and tibial components. The shape of both the femoral and tibial component has become more anatomical, except on the femoral side of mobile bearing designs. An anatomic shape is especially important on the tibial side to maximize capping of the cut surface of the tibial plateau and resist loosening and subsidence.

Finally, in the 2010s, custom patient-specific femoral and tibial components became available to try to accurately replicate each individual patient's anatomy.[9,10] They are coupled with custom patient-specific instruments to aid the surgeon in bone preparation while minimizing the inventory needs of both the prostheses and the implantation instruments.

REFERENCES

1. Gunston FH. Polycentric knee arthroplasty. *Clin Orthop*. 1973;94:128–135.
2. Marmor L. Results of single compartment arthroplasty with acrylic cement fixation. *Clin Orthop*. 1977;122:181–188.
3. Insall J, Walker P. Unicondylar knee replacement. *Clin Orthop*. 1976;120:83–85.
4. Laskin RS. Unicompartmental tibiofemoral resurfacing arthroplasty. *J Bone Joint Surg Am*. 1978;60:182–185.
5. Scott RD, Santore RF. Unicondylar unicompartmental knee replacement in osteoarthritis. *J Bone Joint Surg Am*. 1981;63:536–544.
6. Scott RD, Cobb AG, McQueary FG, Thornhill TS. Unicompartmental knee arthroplasty eight- to twelve-year follow-up evaluation with survivorship analysis. *Clin Orthop*. 1991;271:96–100.
7. Insall JN, Hood RW, Flawn LB, Sullivan DJ. The total condylar knee prosthesis in gonarthrosis: a five- to nine-year follow-up of the first one hundred consecutive replacements. *J Bone Joint Surg Am*. 1983;65:619–628.
8. Scott RD. Robert Brigham unicondylar knee surgical technique. *Tech Orthop*. 1990;5:15–23.
9. Slamin J, Parsley B. Evolution of customization design for total knee arthroplasty. *Curr Rev Musculoskelet Med*. 2012;5(4):290–295.
10. Fitz W. Unicompartmental knee arthroplasty with use of novel patient-specific resurfacing implants and personalized jigs. *J Bone Joint Surg Am*. 2009;91(suppl 1):69–76.

2

Selection Criteria

In theory, unicompartmental knee arthroplasty (UKA) is an attractive alternative to high tibial osteotomy (HTO) and total knee arthroplasty (TKA) in selected osteoarthritic patients. Advantages of UKA over osteotomy include higher initial success, fewer early complications, greater longevity, better cosmetic limb alignment, easier conversion to TKA, and the potential to perform bilateral procedures on the same day. Compared to revision of UKA to TKA, conversion of HTO to TKA is potentially complicated by many factors including the presence of prior incisions, difficult operative exposure, the presence of retained hardware, joint line angle distortion, malunion, nonunion, patella baja, offset tibial shafts, and relative deficiency of the lateral tibial plateau.

Advantages of UKA over TKA include the preservation of both cruciate ligaments, resulting in more normal knee kinematics and the potential for a higher level of performance. Bone stock is preserved in the opposite and patellofemoral compartments, allowing easier conversion to TKA should this be necessary (see Chapter 10). Some initial reports did not confirm that UKA conversion was necessarily an easy procedure.[1] Later reports, however, showed that if the UKA was done in a conservative fashion, conversion was easy and results were the same as those for primary TKA.[2] Most important was a conservative initial resection on the tibial side of the joint (Fig. 2.1).[3] Potential revision problems involved in HTO, TKA, and UKA conversion are listed in Table 2.1. In UKA, the only potential revision problem should be medial tibial plateau deficiency treated with bone graft or metal wedge augmentation if the initial tibial resection was not at a conservative level (Fig. 2.2).

CLASSIC SELECTION CRITERIA

In 1989, Kozinn and Scott reported on the ideal candidate for unicompartmental arthroplasty.[4] Criteria included an elderly patient, noninflammatory osteoarthritis, a mechanical axis deformity of less than 10 degrees of varus or 5 degrees of valgus, an intact anterior cruciate ligament (ACL) without mediolateral subluxation, a flexion contracture less than 15 degrees, a body weight less than 80 to 90 kg, and patellofemoral changes not greater than grade II or III.

Several years later, Stern and colleagues studied their patient population with osteoarthritis and found that 6% of patients fulfilled all these selection criteria.[5] Coincidentally, approximately 6% of the knee arthroplasty market at that time received unicompartmental replacement. This percentage remained relatively stable until the advent of minimally invasive surgery at the beginning of the 21st century.[6] Enthusiasm for the procedure began to grow quickly, perhaps to a point at which some perspective was lost regarding indications for the procedure.

Some surgeons' perspective also changed somewhat when second decade survivorship in unicompartmental devices implanted in the mid-1970s was examined.[7] Although the reoperation rate progressed for the first decade at roughly 1% per year of follow-up, the need for revision surgery appeared to grow faster in the second decade than that seen for bicompartmental replacement performed in the same era. This made some surgeons question the advisability of performing UKA in patients in their 60s and 70s with approximately 15 to 20 years of life expectancy. These patients would have a greater statistical chance of requiring further surgery throughout the remainder of their lifetime with UKA rather than TKA. Using this rationale, some UKA advocates began to stratify UKA candidates into two categories. The first would be a middle-aged patient, especially female, and the second would be an octogenarian (see Chapter 9). A UKA was thought of as the first arthroplasty in middle-aged patients that would buy them 10 or more years of

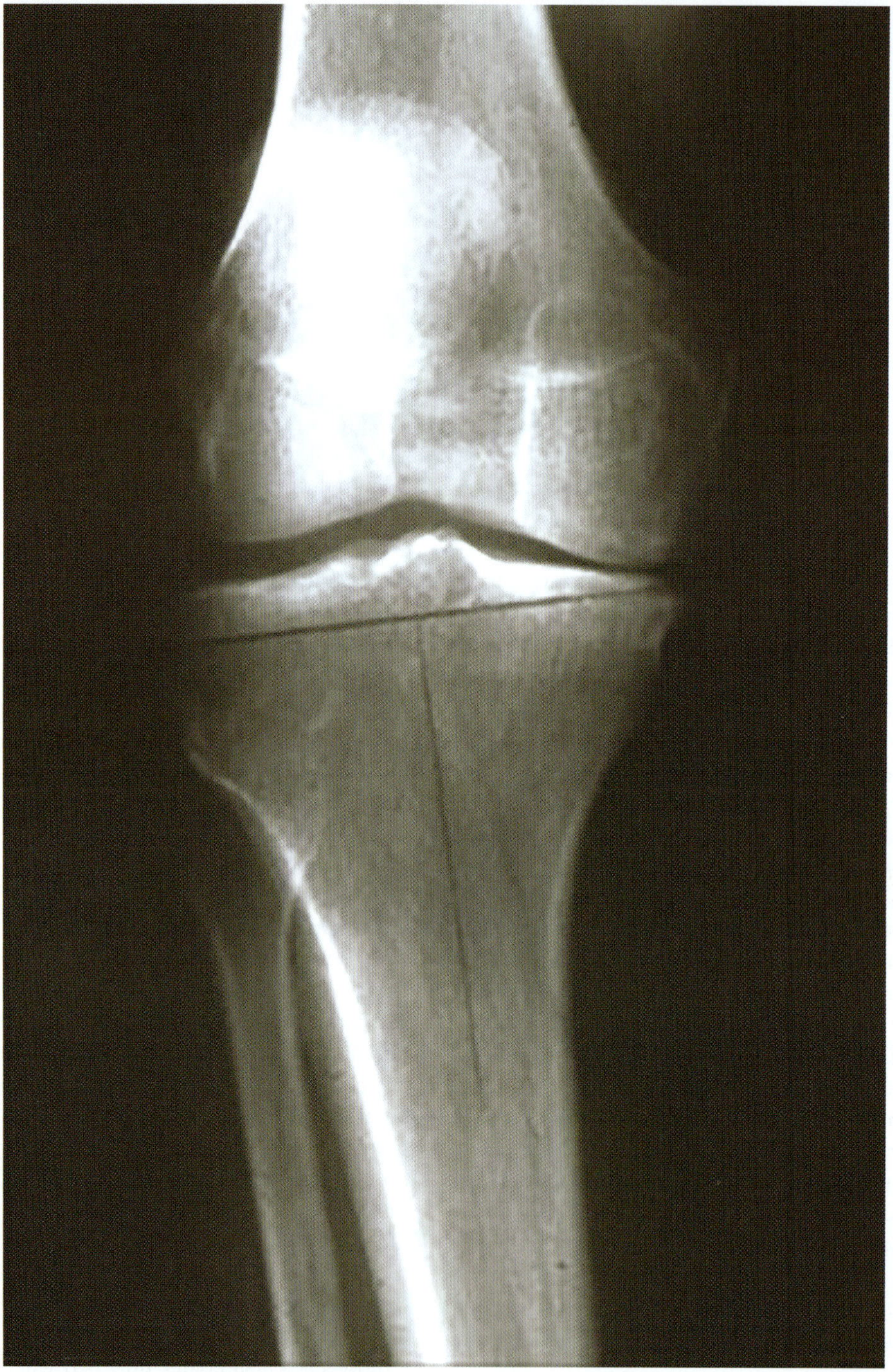

Fig. 2.1 The appropriate initial tibial resection for a unicompartmental knee arthroplasty can be determined by drawing a conservative tibial resection for a total knee arthroplasty on the preoperative radiograph and reproducing the level of the medial resection at the time of the arthroplasty. (From Scott, RD. *Total Knee Arthroplasty*. 2nd ed. Philadelphia: Saunders; 2014).

TABLE 2.1 Revision Problems Seen in Osteotomy, Total Knee Arthroplasty, and Unicompartmental Knee Arthroplasty Conversion

Problems	Tibial Osteotomy	TKA	UKA
Unusable prior incision	+	−	−
Poorly accessible prior hardware	+	−	−
Joint line angle distortion	+/−	+/−	−
Malunion	+/−	−	−
Nonunion	+/−	−	−
Patella baja	+/−	+/−	−
Offset tibial shaft	+/−	−	−
Deficient femoral bone	−	+	−
Deficient patellar bone	−	+	−
Deficient lateral tibial bone	+/−	+	−
Deficient medial tibial bone	+/−	+	+/−

TKA, Total knee arthroplasty; *UKA,* unicompartmental knee arthroplasty.

longevity with an easy conversion to TKA when that was inevitably necessary in later life. They would benefit from a high initial success, few early complications and an acceptable cosmetic appearance relative to HTO, preservation of both cruciate ligaments relative to TKA, and an easier revision in comparison with both HTO and TKA.

Advantages for the octogenarian would include faster recovery, less blood loss, less medical morbidity, and a less expensive procedure to be borne by the health care system. Given the life expectancy and activity level of octogenarians, the UKA would be unlikely to require revision in their lifetime.[8]

The indications and contraindications for lateral UKA are similar to those for medial replacement. Patients with isolated lateral disease, however, are more likely to have an inflammatory synovitis (a contraindication) associated with chondrocalcinosis (see Chapter 8). In addition, they are more likely to have significant patellofemoral disease that may contraindicate the procedure. An additional contraindication specific to lateral UKA is attenuation of the medial collateral ligament (Fig. 2.3).

CONTEMPORARY SELECTION CRITERIA

Recently, improvements in prosthetic design and surgical technique have led to revision of the classic selection criteria for medial compartment arthroplasty (described by Kozinn and Scott[4]) to ones that are much more liberal.[9] In 2015, six arthroplasty surgeons from the United States and Europe with a combined experience of performing over 8000 unicompartmental replacements were surveyed and a consensus for updated indications and contraindications for the procedure was formulated. The use of UKA in each practice varied from 10% to 50%. Each surgeon independently listed their current indications and contraindications and was asked to provide peer-reviewed published references to support their opinion. Discussion ensued, a new proposal was formulated and then redistributed for final modification in order to address any individual concerns.

The consensus basically confirmed the Kozinn and Scott criteria but removed some of the contraindications to the procedure. The primary indication for medial UKA remains grade IV anteromedial osteoarthritis (bone on bone) or greater than 95% loss of medial compartment joint space on a standing anteroposterior (AP) or 30- to 45-degree posteroanterior (PA) flexed radiograph. It was noted that the lateral compartment should have less than 25% loss of joint space on a stress radiograph and confirmed to be essentially normal on direct inspection at arthrotomy. Some lateral spurring is acceptable.

Avascular necrosis (osteonecrosis) isolated to the medial compartment was added as a secondary indication for medial UKA. It was noted that magnetic resonance imaging may be useful in defining that the disease is localized.

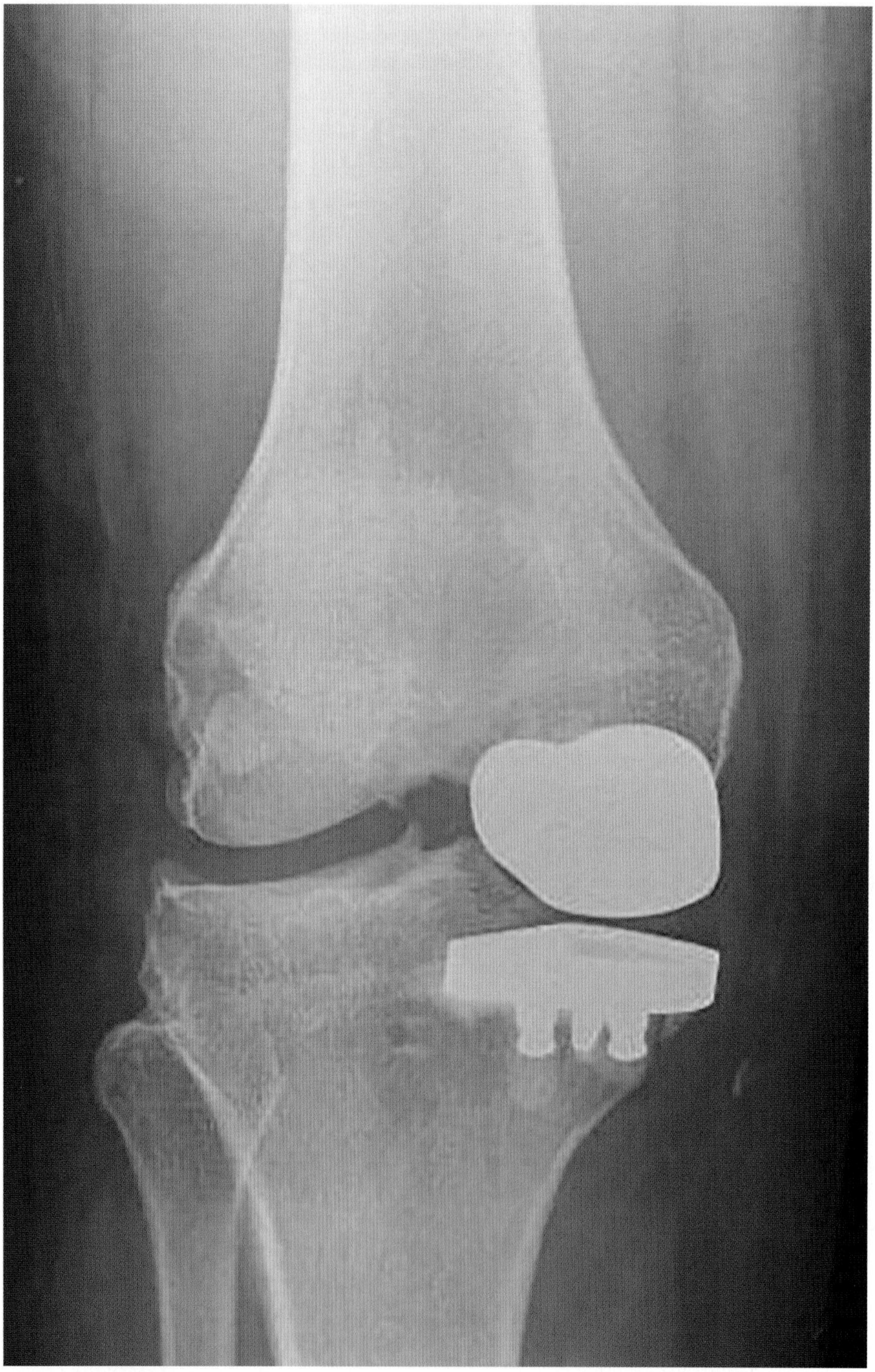

Fig. 2.2 This excessive tibial resection will require significant medial augmentation and a long-stem tibial component at the time of revision.

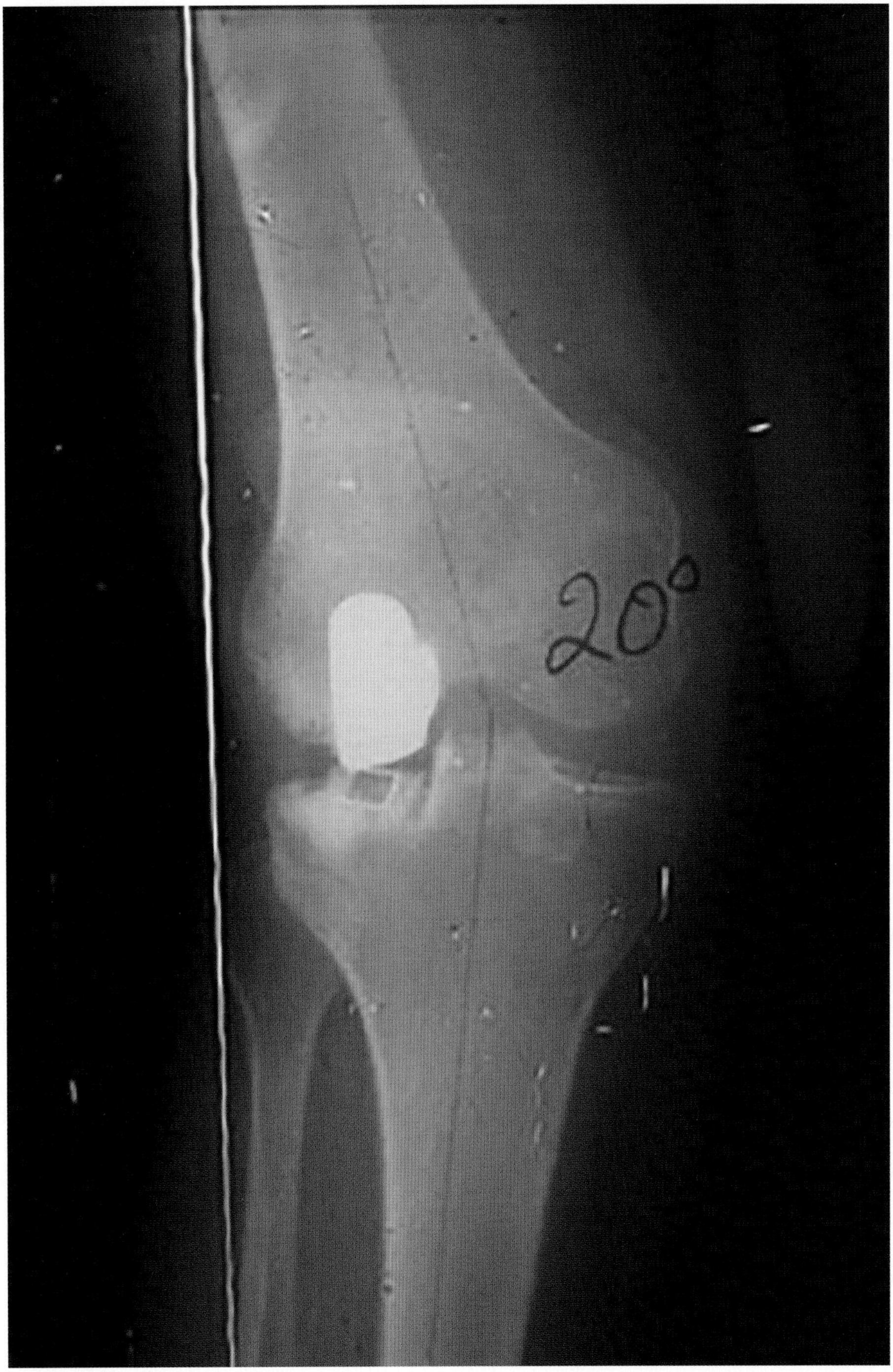

Fig. 2.3 Unicompartmental knee arthroplasty failed to restore stability to this severe valgus knee with medial collateral ligament laxity.

Importantly, some contraindications were removed or modified. Obesity with a body mass index (BMI) over 32 may no longer be a contraindication to UKA as long as a metal-backed tibial component is utilized. Modern metal-backed components whether fixed- or mobile-bearing have been reported to fare well in the obese.[10,11] Relatively young age was also no longer considered a contraindication but caution was expressed that young patients tend to have higher expectations and when revisions occur, they are often triggered by the presence of unexplained pain. It was emphasized that UKA remains an attractive first conservative arthroplasty in this age group and that a conservative initial tibial resection is important.

The significance of patellofemoral disease was reexamined. All agreed that in medial arthroplasty, grade IV changes on the lateral side of the patella or trochlea were contraindications. Three of the six surgeons, however, would accept these changes if they were confined to the medial patellofemoral articulation. Radiographic chondrocalcinosis by itself was not a contraindication unless accompanied by inflammatory synovitis.

Prior HTO was considered a contraindication unless the osteotomy failed with residual varus or neutral tibiofemoral alignment. An osteotomy healed in any degree of anatomic valgus was not an appropriate UKA candidate.

The status of the ACL remains of importance (see Chapter 9). Most mobile-bearing advocates feel that an absent ACL is an absolute contraindication to UKA using a mobile-bearing articulation for fear of bearing subluxation. Others may still employ a mobile-bearing if a concomitant ACL reconstruction can be accomplished that restores anterior-posterior stability. Fixed-bearing advocates will often make a decision about the feasibility of UKA in a compromised ACL depending on the tibial wear pattern. In classic varus-aligned medial compartment arthritis, the initial tibial wear pattern is anteromedial.[12] As ACL insufficiency ensues, the wear pattern moves posteriorly. If the wear pattern is central, fixed bearing UKA is appropriate. If the wear pattern has become posterior, any form of UKA is contraindicated unless corrected by an ACL reconstruction.

REFERENCES

1. Barrett WP, Scott RD. Revision of failed unicondylar unicompartmental knee arthroplasty. *J Bone Joint Surg Am.* 1987;69:1328–1335.
2. Levine WN, Ozuna RM, Scott RD, Thornhill TS. Conversion of failed modern unicompartmental arthroplasty to total knee arthroplasty. *J Arthroplasty.* 1996;11:797–801.
3. Schwarzkopf R, Mikhael B, Li L, Josephs L, Scott RD. Effect of initial tibial resection thickness on outcomes of revision UKA. *Orthopedics.* 2013;36(4):409–414.
4. Kozinn SC, Scott RD. Unicondylar knee arthroplasty: current concepts review. *J Bone Joint Surg Am.* 1989;71:145–150.
5. Stern SH, Becker MW, Insall JN. Unicondylar knee arthroplasty: an evaluation of selection criteria. *Clin Orthop.* 1993;286:143–148.
6. Repicci JA, Hartman JF. Minimally invasive unicondylar knee arthroplasty for the treatment of unicompartmental osteoarthritis: an outpatient arthritic bypass procedure. *Orthop Clin North Am.* 2004;35:201–216.
7. Scott RD, Cobb AG, McQueary FG, Thornhill TS. Unicompartmental knee arthroplasty eight- to twelve-year follow-up evaluation with survivorship analysis. *Clin Orthop.* 1991;271:96–100.
8. Sah AP, Springer BD, Scott RD. Unicompartmental knee arthroplasty in octogenarians: survival longer than the patient. *Clin Orthop.* 2006;4:107–112.
9. Berend KR, Berend ME, Dalury DF, Argenson JN, Dodd CA, Scott RD. Consensus statement on indications and contraindications for medial unicompartmental knee arthroplasty. *J Surg Orthop Adv.* 2015;24(4):252–256.
10. Murray DW, Pandit H, Weston-Simons JS, et al. Does body mass index affect the outcome of unicompartmental knee replacement? *Knee.* 2013;20(6):461–465.
11. Cavaignac E, Lafontan V, Reina N, et al. Obesity has no adverse effect on the outcomes of unicompartmental knee replacement at a minimum follow-up of seven years. *Bone Joint J.* 2013;95B(8):1064–1068.
12. White SH, Ludkowski PF, Goodfellow JW. Anteromedial osteoarthritis of the knee. *J Bone Joint Surg Br.* 1991;73:582–586.

3

Prosthetic Design Considerations

Unicompartmental components have been available for over 50 years, beginning with designs such as the Polycentric Knee, and the Marmor Knee prostheses.[1,2] Many of these early designs were also advocated for bicompartmental arthroplasty, but their success was hindered by the fact that instrumentation was poor and they did not provide for resurfacing of the patellofemoral compartment. As time passed, one-piece bicompartmental components became available on both the femoral and tibial sides and femoral components eventually had trochlear flanges to allow for resurfacing of the patellofemoral compartment. From that point, the use of individual components for each condyle and plateau has been mostly confined to unicompartmental arthroplasty of either the medial or lateral compartment. There is some limited experience combining medial or lateral unicompartmental components with modular patellofemoral components.

Experience has shown that certain design features of either the femoral or tibial component can favor ease of implantation, conservation of bone stock, and longevity of the arthroplasty. These features include size options, prosthetic geometry, symmetry versus asymmetry, primary fixation (cement versus ingrowth), and ancillary fixation (keels and lugs).

THE FEMORAL COMPONENT

Sizing

Early designs often provided just two sizes: large and small. Since the early 2000s, size options for fixed-bearing femoral components have increased to as many as five. The advantage of multiple sizes is the ease of accommodating extremes of size variation, but disadvantages include inventory management problems. The advent of custom patient-specific components addresses both size variation and inventory issues[3,4] (see Chapter 11).

Prosthetic Geometry

The sagittal shape of the femoral component should attempt to replicate the radius of curvature of the native distal femoral condyle. It must also allow for adequate capping of the resected surface of the posterior condyle. Most components call for a linear resection of the posterior condyle to facilitate bone preparation (Fig. 3.1). Where "robotic" bone preparation is utilized, nonlinear resection can be appropriate. The sagittal femoral component shape must also allow adequate recession of the leading edge of the component in order to eliminate the potential for patellar impingement as the knee goes into flexion.

From a coronal perspective, the articulating surface of the femoral component should have a radius of curvature that is large but not infinite (flat) in order to allow for adequate contact between the femoral and tibial articular surfaces. Flat on round articulations are never appropriate. Flat on flat articulations are prone to edge-loading (see Fig. 1.4). Round on round articulations cannot be fully congruent unless they are mobile-bearing (see later). Round on relatively flat (large radius of curvature) articulations are appropriate as long as the polyethylene is of high quality and wear resistant. The coronal width of the femoral component should be proportional to the sagittal sizing and wide enough to adequately cap the prepared surface of the femur and resist subsidence (see Figs. 1.1 and 1.2).

For a cemented femoral component, the surface that contacts bone should promote cement fixation and containment, most often achieved via cement "pockets." For cementless fixation, a surface that encourages bone ingrowth is required.

Symmetry versus Asymmetry

Early designs were symmetric and could be used on either condyle and in both right and left knees. All modern

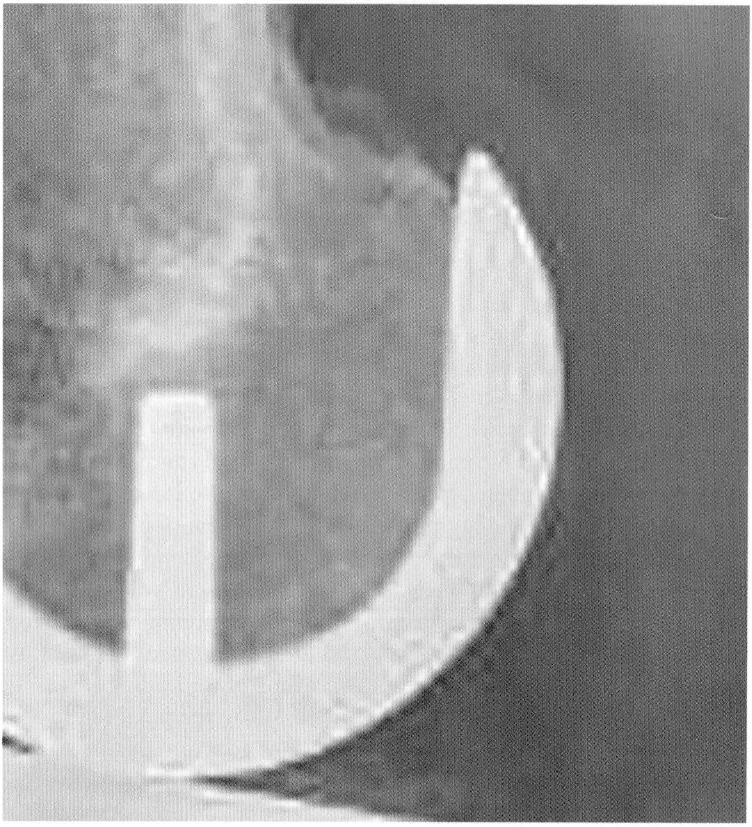

Fig. 3.1 A Radiograph Showing a Linear Posterior Condylar Resection.

designs, except for mobile-bearing articulations, are asymmetric to better conform to patient anatomy. Very few systems provide separate femoral component designs for the medial and lateral condyles and rely on the availability of multiple sizes to accommodate the slightly smaller lateral condyle. Custom components, of course, will provide the most accurate replication of a patient's anatomy.

Primary Fixation

Cement has been traditionally used for component fixation with great success. Components are available in some systems for cementless use with bone ingrowth potential and some encouraging early results.[5,6] Long-term longevity has yet to be determined. A possible argument against cementless fixation is the need for condylar resection to be deep enough to allow bone ingrowth. Furthermore, if fixation is dependent on ingrowth into deeply penetrating lugs or fins, extraction of well-fixed components could lead to significant loss of bone stock.

Ancillary Fixation

Ancillary fixation, whether in cemented or cementless components, is achieved via lugs, keels, or a combination of both. When fins are utilized, they must be relatively narrow and not so deep as to cause loss of bone stock upon removal. Lugs can be round in cross section or square and also vary in length with the same caveat that longer lugs will risk loss of bone upon removal. They are often slightly conical in the sagittal view and can be tapered, smooth, rough, porous, or corrugated, depending on whether they are used with or without cement (Fig. 3.2). Lugs should probably be angled away from and not parallel to a linear posterior condylar resection in order to achieve maximum prosthesis to bone contact upon insertion (Fig. 3.3).

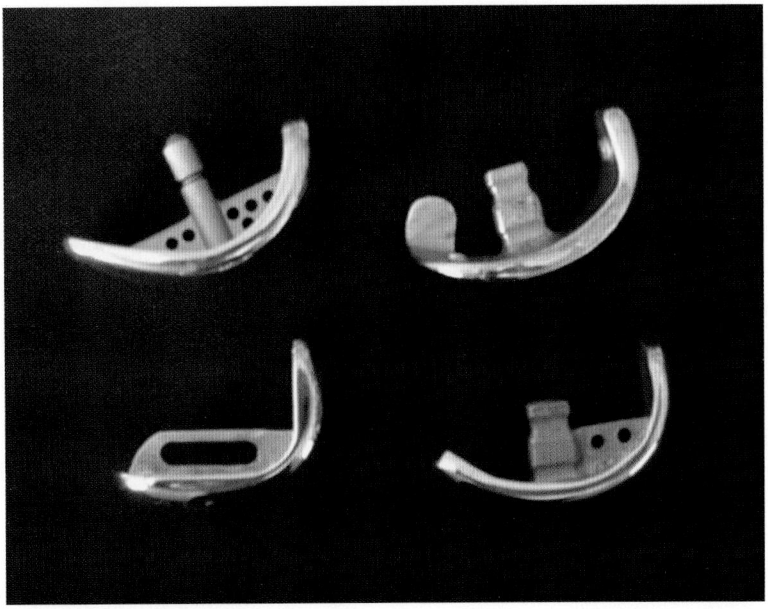

Fig. 3.2 Examples of Modes of Ancillary Femoral Component Fixation Via Lugs and Keels.

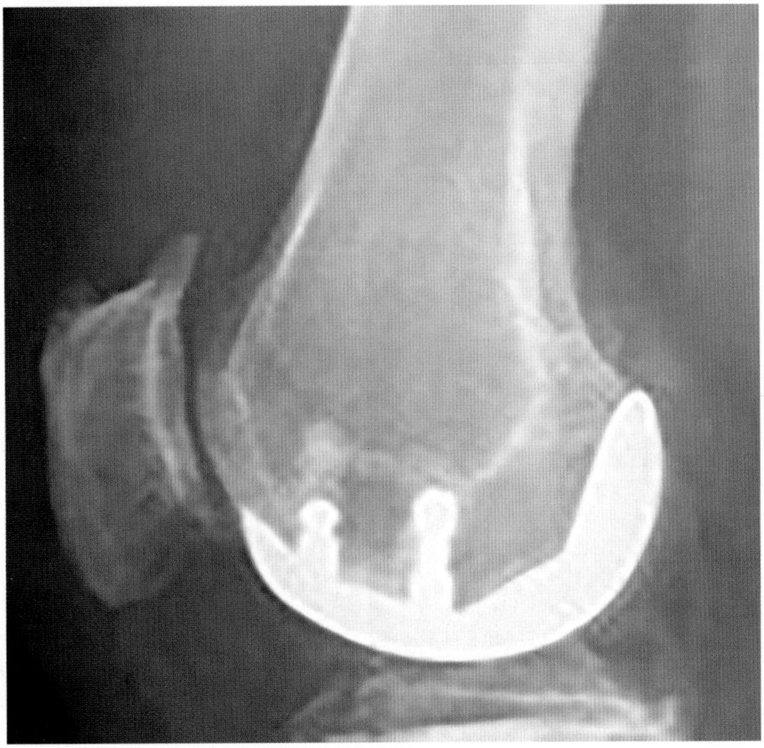

Fig. 3.3 Lugs that diverge away from the posterior condylar resection allow pressurization of the posterior prosthesis to bone interface during insertion.

Keels can be of various depths and thicknesses as well as smooth or porous (when used cementless). The deeper they are, the more loss of bone stock can occur upon removal. They also increase the risk of femoral condylar fracture during bone preparation and component insertion or removal. For this reason, shallow keels are probably preferable.

THE TIBIAL COMPONENT

Sizing

Similar to the femoral component, early designs often provided just two sizes: large and small. Since the early 2000s, size options for fixed-bearing tibial components have also increased to as many as five with the same advantages and disadvantages noted previously on the femoral side. Again, custom components address the disadvantages.

Prosthetic Geometry

Two types of tibial components have been available. One is referred to as "on-lay" and the other as "inset" or "in-lay" (Figs. 3.4 and 3.5). The on-lay component attempts to maximally cap the cut surface of the tibia that is prepared by a reciprocating saw, whereas the inset component preserves peripheral bone and is in-laid by a milling process, sometimes with the use of a robot. The shape of the on-lay tibial component should come close to replicating the outline of the resected tibial bone it replaces, so that it maximally caps the cut surface while avoiding component overhang. This will minimize the chance for component subsidence or loosening. The inset component will also benefit from maximally capping the proximal tibial bone available for the milling process. On-lay components were originally symmetric to save inventory by allowing use in right and left medial and lateral compartments, but most designs are now more anatomic in shape for maximum capping of the resected bone.

The lateral compartment has a different proportional shape than the medial compartment, being shorter in the anterior-posterior (AP) dimension relative to the medial-lateral (ML) dimension. This is usually addressed in off-the-shelf components by utilizing the largest size component that does not overhang bone in the AP dimension. Some implant companies are beginning to address this issue with separate lateral tibial components at the expense of increasing inventory. Custom components, of course, can address this size issue more precisely.

Modularity

Initially, in the 1970s, tibial components were all-polyethylene. As metal-backing was shown to be favorable in terms of stress transmission to underlying bone, the option of having a modular component also became attractive in terms of inventory management, intraoperative flexibility, and possible revision options for wear or instability. For decades, however, a requirement that

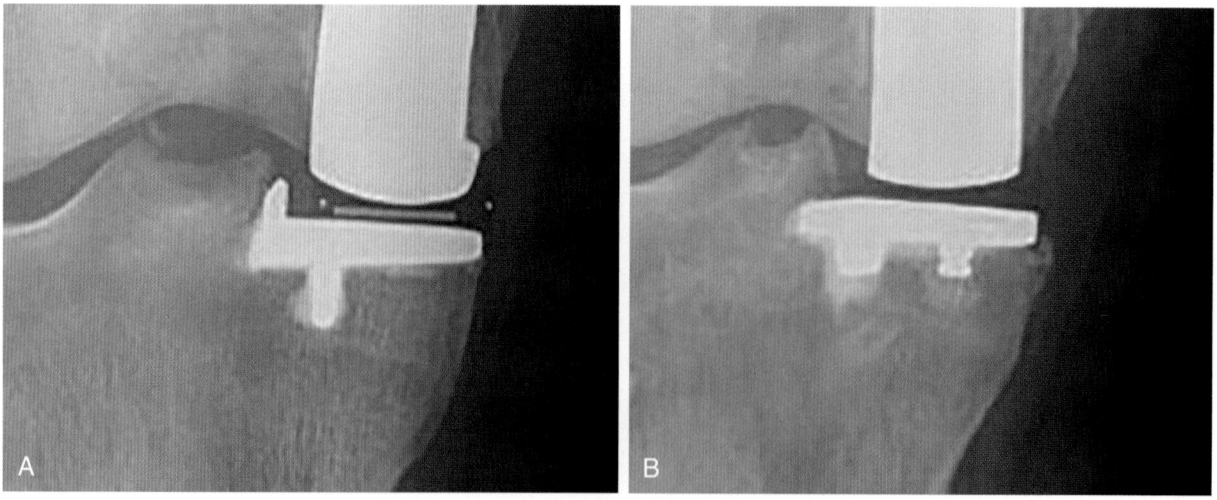

Fig. 3.4 (A) An example of an on-lay tibial component with ancillary keel fixation. (B) An example of an on-lay tibial component with a combination of a keel and an anterior lug.

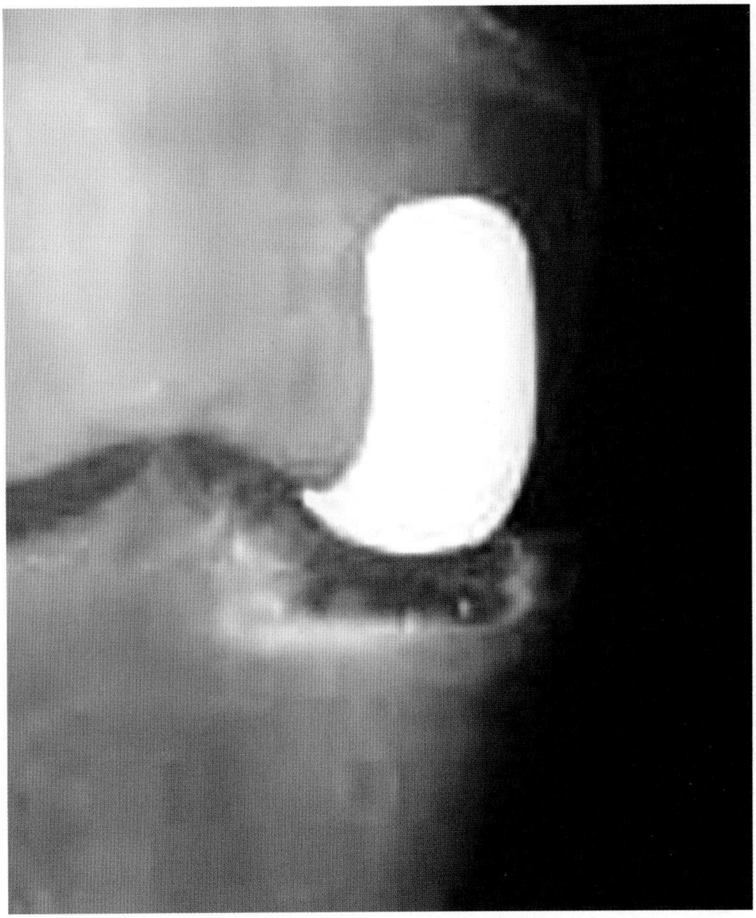

Fig. 3.5 A Radiograph Showing an Implanted Inset All-Polyethylene Tibial Component.

articulating polyethylene have a minimum thickness of 6 mm meant that composite component thickness (polyethylene plus metal) was 9 or 10 mm. This detracted from the conservative goal of unicompartmental arthroplasty. Improvements in polyethylene and metallurgy have allowed minimum composite thicknesses as small as 7 mm in fixed-bearing designs and 6 mm in mobile-bearing tibial components.

Articulating Geometry

From a coronal perspective, the articulating surface of the tibial polyethylene should have a radius of curvature that is large and even approach infinite (flat) as long as the femoral component coronal geometry has a smaller radius of curvature and minimizes the possibility of significant edge-loading in well-aligned components. The exception is in the mobile-bearing design where similar radii of curvature are both acceptable and encouraged to maximize polyethylene wear.[7,8]

From a sagittal perspective, a fixed-bearing component must also have a very large (almost flat) radius of curvature. The classic wear pattern in medial unicompartmental osteoarthritis is anterior and peripheral[9] (Fig. 3.6A). The arthroplasty articulation wants to return to this preoperative wear pattern[10] (Fig. 3.6B). Attempts to control this wear pattern with a conforming fixed-bearing arthroplasty have led to an increased incidence of component loosening.[11] It is also important to remember that metal-backed tibial components, whether modular or not, require adequate thickness of polyethylene to be maintained in the anterior aspect of the articulation. As noted earlier with coronal geometry, mobile-bearing sagittal

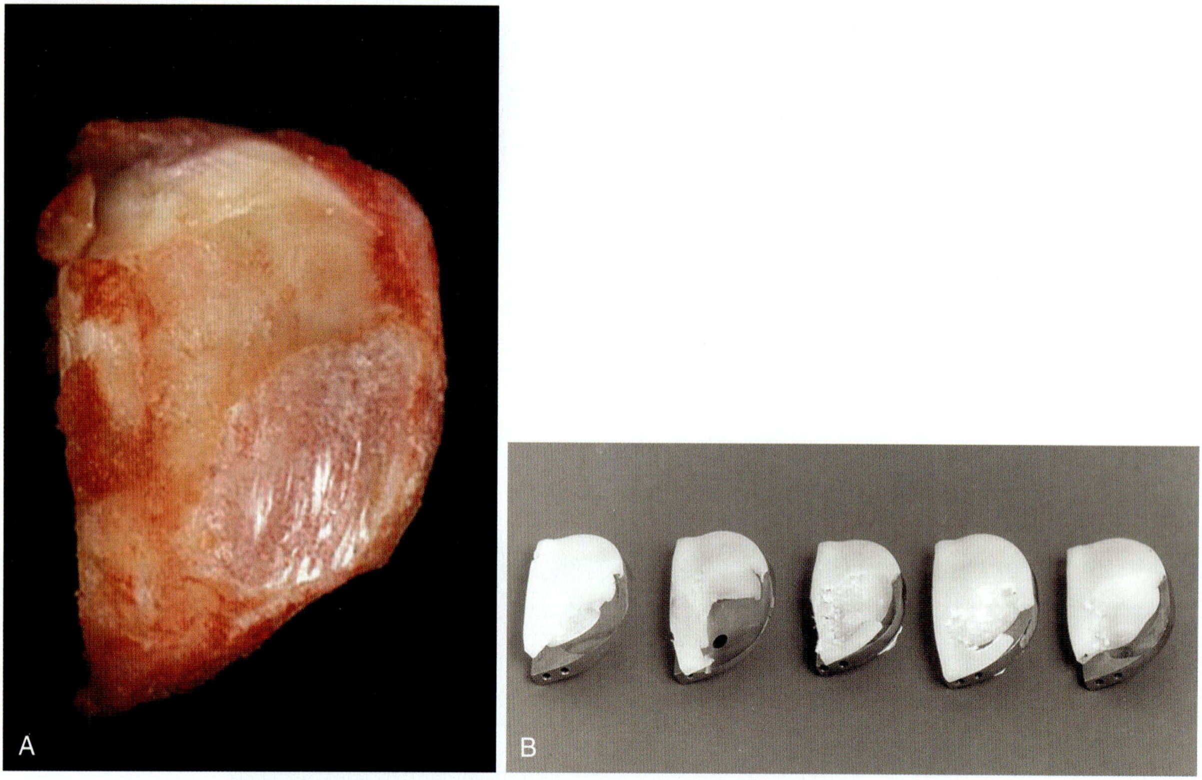

Fig 3.6 (A) A resected specimen showing the classic anteromedial wear pattern in medial osteoarthritis. (B) Retrieved failed metal-backed tibial components all showing a return to an anteromedial wear pattern and resultant wear-through of thin anterior polyethylene.

geometry can be very conforming to maximize polyethylene wear without adverse effects on component fixation.

Primary Fixation

As on the femoral side, cement has been traditionally used for component fixation with great success. Components are available in some systems for cementless use with bone ingrowth potential with some encouraging early results.[5,6] Long-term longevity has yet to be determined. A possible argument against cementless fixation is the need for tibial resection to be deep enough to allow bone ingrowth.

Ancillary Fixation

Ancillary fixation (whether in cemented or cementless components) is achieved via lugs, keels, or a combination of both (see Fig. 3.4). When keels are utilized, they must be relatively narrow and not so deep as to cause loss of bone stock upon removal. Lugs can be round in cross section or square and also vary in length with the caveat that longer posterior lugs can be difficult to insert due to the limited posterior tibial exposure available in unicompartmental arthroplasty. Lugs can be rough, porous, or corrugated, depending on whether they are used with or without cement.

Keels can be of various depths and thicknesses as well as smooth, rough, or porous (when used cementless). The deeper they are, the more loss of bone stock can occur upon removal. Insertion of a keel is not limited by exposure. For this reason, some systems advocate an anterior lug and a posterior keel combination (see Fig. 3.4B).

MOBILE-BEARING COMPONENT DESIGN

Femoral

Sizing

Because of the nature of a mobile-bearing articulation advocating maximum articulating congruency between the femoral and tibial components, femoral components have a spherical sagittal shape that permits fewer sizes. The spherical shape does not allow anatomic capping at the anterior aspect of the femoral component. Instead the leading edge is recessed into the bone to prevent patellar impingement (Fig. 3.7).

Prosthetic Geometry

As noted earlier, the outer sagittal geometry is spherical with a continuous radius of curvature. The inner geometry also remains spherical with the bone prepared and shaped with reamers. The posterior condylar preparation can be linear by way of a reciprocating saw (see Chapter 7).

The coronal articulating geometry is also spherical to allow maximum congruency with the mobile polyethylene bearing that in turn articulates on a polished tibial tray.

Symmetry versus Asymmetry

Mobile-bearing femoral components are symmetrical and can be used on either condyle in both right and left knees. When used in the lateral compartment, however, they are usually meant to articulate with a fixed-bearing

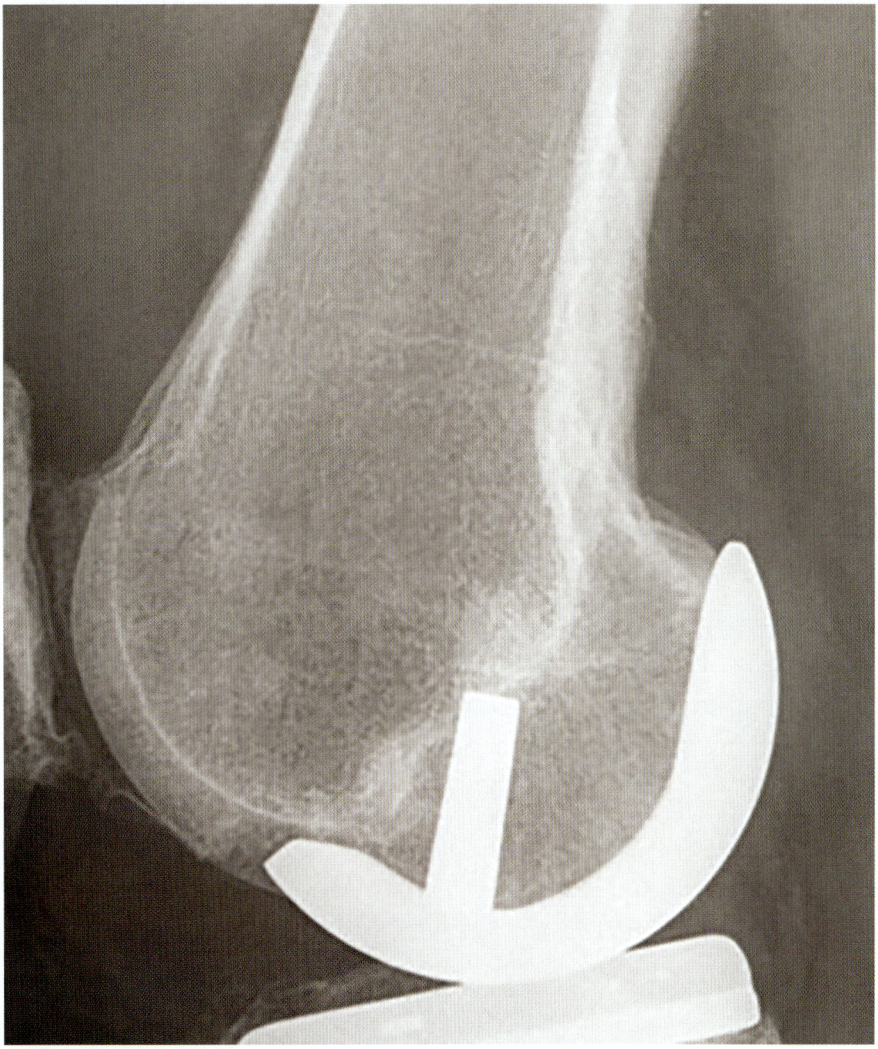

Fig. 3.7 A lateral radiograph of a mobile-bearing unicompartmental knee arthroplasty showing the surgically created anterior femoral recession to alleviate potential impingement of the tibial polyethylene in full knee extension.

tibial component because of concerns of potential posterior bearing subluxation with excessive roll-back in high knee flexion.

Primary and Ancillary Fixation

The aspects of primary and ancillary fixation are similar to those described previously for fixed-bearing components.

REFERENCES

1. Gunston FH. Polycentric knee arthroplasty. *Clin Orthop*. 1973;94:128–135.
2. Marmor L. Results of single compartment arthroplasty with acrylic cement fixation. *Clin Orthop*. 1977;122:181–188.
3. Slamin J, Parsley B. Evolution of customization design for total knee arthroplasty. *Curr Rev Musculoskelet Med*. 2012;5(4):290–295.
4. Fitz W. Unicompartmental knee arthroplasty with use of novel patient-specific resurfacing implants and personalized jigs. *J Bone Joint Surg Am*. 2009;91(suppl 1):69–76.
5. Stempin R, Stempin K, Kaczmarek W. Medium-term outcome of cementless, mobile-bearing, unicompartmental knee arthroplasty. *Ann Transl Med*. 2019;7(3):41.
6. Campi S, Pandit H, Hooper G, et al. Ten-year survival and seven-year functional results of cementless Oxford unicompartmental knee replacement: a prospective consecutive series of our first 1000 cases. *Knee*. 2018; 25(6):1231–1237.
7. Goodfellow J, O'Connor J, Murray DW. The Oxford meniscal unicompartmental knee. *J Knee Surg*. 2002;15:240–246.
8. Mohammad HR, Strickland L, Hamilton TW, Murray DW. Long-term outcomes of over 8,000 medial Oxford phase 3 unicompartmental knees-a systematic review. *Acta Orthop*. 2018;89(1):101–107.
9. White SH, Ludkowski PF, Goodfellow JW. Anteromedial osteoarthritis of the knee. *J Bone Joint Surg Br*. 1991;73: 582–586.
10. McCallum JD, Scott RD. Duplication of medial erosion in unicompartmental knee arthroplasties. *J Bone Joint Surg Br*. 1995;77:726–728.
11. Scott RD. Three decades of experience with unicompartmental knee arthroplasty: mistakes made and lessons learned. *Orthopedics*. 2006;29(9):829–831.

4

Reasons for and Modes of Failure of Unicompartmental Knee Arthroplasty

Reasons for failure of unicompartmental knee arthroplasty (UKA) include improper patient selection, poor prosthetic design, improper surgical technique, and pain of unknown origin. Modes of failure include prosthetic loosening and wear, secondary degeneration of an unresurfaced compartment, instability, and stress fracture of the tibia through peripherally placed guide pins.

IMPROPER PATIENT SELECTION

The "classic" and updated guidelines for appropriate patient selection are given in Chapter 2.[1,2] Some controversy still exists regarding patient selection and it is expected that these criteria will slowly continue to evolve.

The original patient selection criteria as espoused by Kozinn and Scott[1] recommended that patients weighing over 80 to 90 kg (176–198 pounds) were not good candidates for UKA for fear of component loosening or subsidence. The criteria were developed when component design was early in its evolution before components of more sizes were made available to better distribute forces across the fixation interface. Failure due to loosening in obese patients has become less frequent,[3,4] although some recent studies still report higher failure rates in the obese population.[5,6] Perhaps more relevant than actual patient body weight predisposing failure is their specific age, gender, and activity level. Mesomorphic middle-aged males appear to be at higher risk for component loosening[2] (see Chapter 9).

POOR PROSTHETIC DESIGN

The effects of poor prosthetic design on the propensity for failure are discussed in Chapter 3. They are mainly due to poor sizing and capping of the available bone, poor fixation, poor articular contact area, poor polyethylene, and excessive articular congruency in fixed bearings. Instrumentation that is insufficient to allow for accurate component implantation can also be a cause of subsequent failure. These effects, of course, will be a less prevalent cause of failure with modern designs and materials.

IMPROPER SURGICAL TECHNIQUE

A unicompartmental arthroplasty is a technically more challenging procedure than a total knee arthroplasty (TKA). The unresurfaced compartments must remain unaffected by the arthroplasty regarding their congruency and balancing. For decades, UKA was only performed in approximately 6% of knee arthroplasties[7] and only more recently has this percentage grown to 10% to 15%. More UKAs are performed in practices with a lot of experience and specialization (as much as 80%), whereas conversely, some surgeons never even consider this option.

Technical errors include overcorrection, undercorrection, component incongruency, patellar impingement, peripheral placement of guide pins, and cement retention. Strategies to avoid these errors are enumerated and illustrated in Chapter 6.

PAIN OF UNKNOWN ORIGIN

Pain of unknown origin in a UKA is not a rare reason for revision.[8] In these cases, radiographs do not show an obvious cause for the patient's complaints and at surgery, a definitive cause is often not determined. Because a UKA has two unresurfaced compartments, surgeons are more likely to recommend revision in these cases, especially if they are not a proponent of the procedure and have no experience with it. Conversely, in a TKA, patient revision is less likely to be recommended when the reason for failure is unknown.

PROSTHETIC LOOSENING AND WEAR

These problems have become less frequent over time as prosthetic design has evolved along with improvements in surgical technique, articular geometry, and polyethylene. Despite being less frequent, however, tibial component loosening is still a major reason for UKA failure. (See Chapters 6 and 7 for details on the role of surgical technique in minimizing late complications.)

SECONDARY DEGENERATION OF AN UNRESURFACED COMPARTMENT

This is usually a late complication. When the opposite compartment deteriorates, the cause can merely be the "normal" progression of an osteoarthritic condition in a well-executed arthroplasty (Fig. 4.1), or the late appearance of an inflammatory component to the patient's disease. For example, a patient may have a diagnosis of pseudogout (chondrocalcinosis) that was quiescent at the time of arthroplasty, but subsequently flared into a chronic condition. An occult diagnosis of rheumatoid arthritis may also become active.

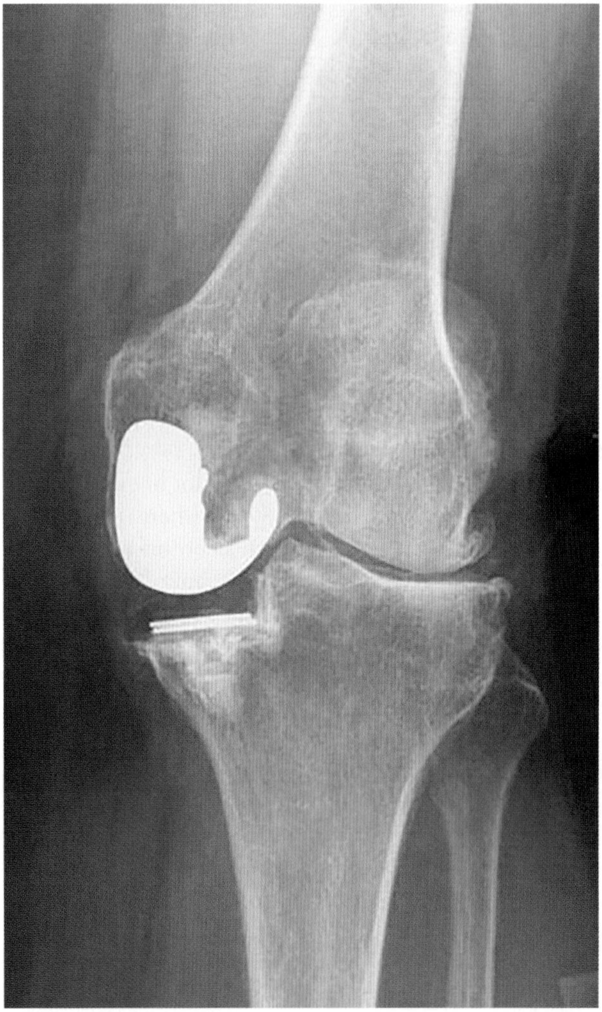

Fig. 4.1 A radiograph taken 24 years after medial unicompartmental knee arthroplasty showing failure due to secondary degeneration of the unresurfaced lateral compartment.

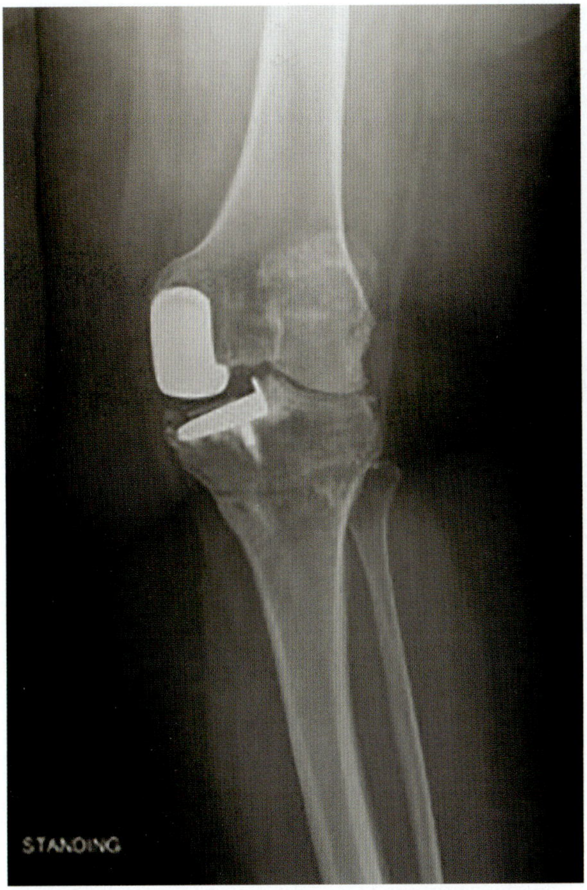

Fig. 4.2 A radiograph of an overcorrected unicompartmental knee arthroplasty.

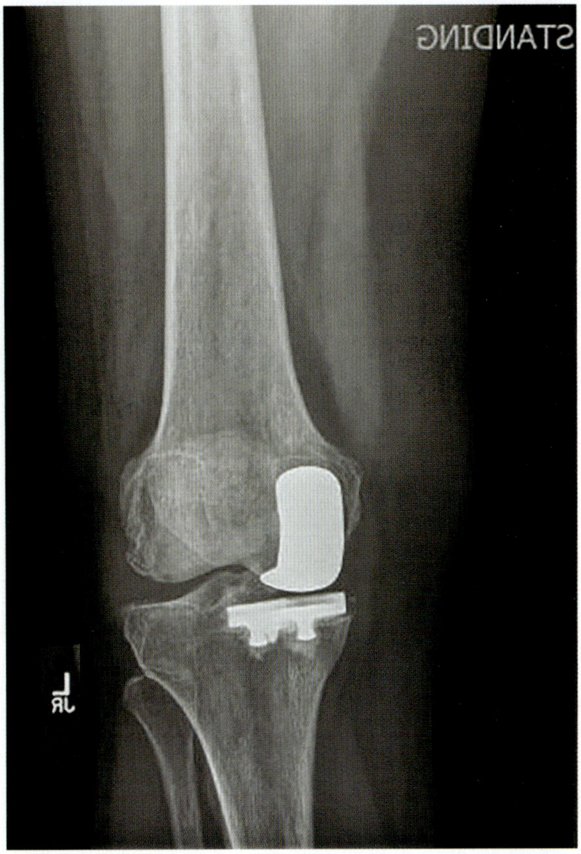

Fig. 4.3 A radiograph of an undercorrected unicompartmental knee arthroplasty with instability because the medial collateral ligament tension was never restored.

More often, however, secondary degeneration of the opposite compartment occurs in the face of overcorrection of the patient's alignment (Fig. 4.2).

INSTABILITY

Failure of a UKA because of instability is almost always an early complication requiring early revision (Fig. 4.3). It is most likely present at the completion of the arthroplasty, but unrecognized until the patient is undergoing their recovery.

TIBIAL STRESS FRACTURE

This complication is avoidable and is most likely the result of a surgically introduced tibial stress riser at the time of the arthroplasty via a peripheral guide pin for a cutting block[9] (Fig. 4.4).

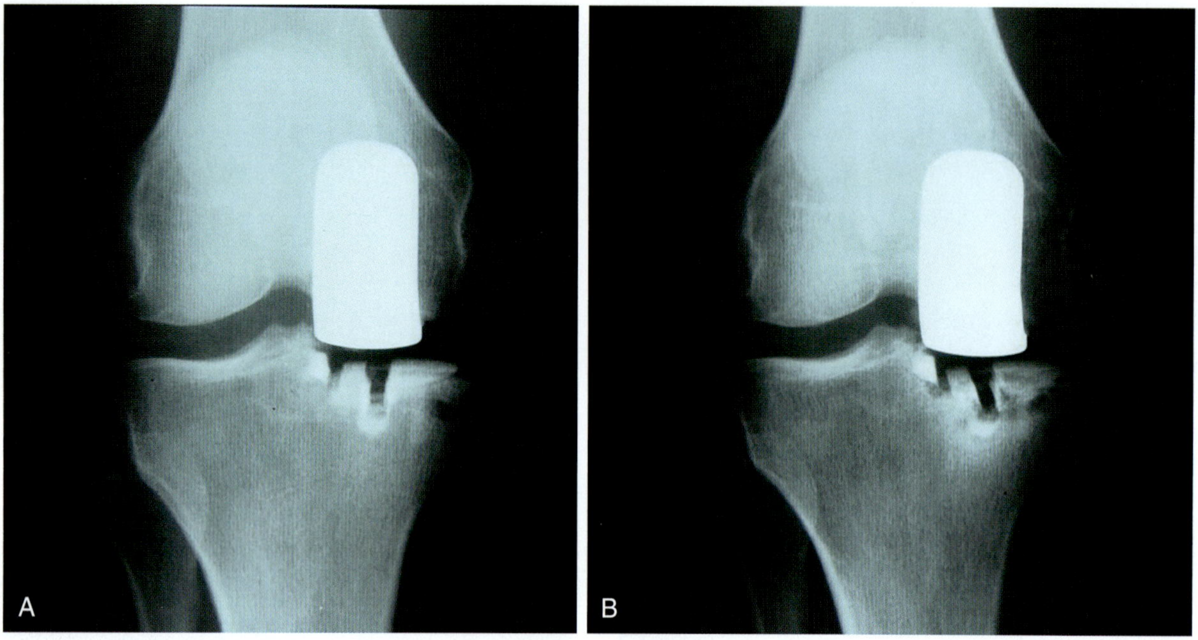

Fig. 4.4 (A) An immediate postoperative radiograph showing a peripheral hole in the proximal tibia where a pin for a cutting guide had been placed at surgery. (B) A radiograph taken several weeks after surgery when the patient presented with a stress fracture through the guide pin hole.

REFERENCES

1. Kozinn SC, Scott RD. Unicondylar knee arthroplasty: current concepts review. *J Bone Joint Surg Am*. 1989;71:145–150.
2. Berend KR, Berend ME, Dalury DF, Argenson J, Dodd CA, Scott RD. Consensus statement on indications and contraindications for medial unicompartmental knee arthroplasty. *J Surg Orthop Adv*. 2015;24(4):252–256.
3. Molloy J, Kennedy J, Jenkins C, Mellon S, Dodd C, Murray D. Obesity should not be considered a contraindication to medial Oxford UKA: long-term patient-reported outcomes and implant survival in 1000 knees. *Knee Surg Sports Traumatol Arthrosc*. 2019;27(7):2259–2265.
4. Cavaignac E, Lafontan V, Reina N, et al. Obesity has no adverse effect on the outcome of unicompartmental knee replacement at a minimum follow-up of seven years. *Bone Joint J*. 2013;95-B(8):1064–1068.
5. Nettrour JF, Ellis RT, Hansen BJ, Keeney JA. High failure rates for unicompartmental knee arthroplasty in morbidly obese patients: a two-year minimum follow-up study. *J Arthroplasty*. 2020;35(4):989–996.
6. Kandil A, Werner BC, Gwathmey WF, Browne JA. Obesity, morbid obesity and their related medical comorbidities are associated with increased complications and revision rates after unicompartmental knee arthroplasty. *J Arthroplasty*. 2015;30(3):456–460.
7. Stern SH, Becker MW, Insall JN. Unicondylar knee arthroplasty: an evaluation of selection criteria. *Clin Orthop*. 1993;286:143–148.
8. El-Galaly A, Kappel A, Nielsen PT, Jensen SL. Revision risk for total knee arthroplasty converted from medial unicompartmental knee arthroplasty: comparison with primary and revision arthroplasties, based on mid-term results from the Danish Knee Arthroplasty Registry. *J Bone Joint Surg Am*. 2019;101(22):1999–2006.
9. Brumby SA, Carrington R, Zayontz S, Reish T, Scott RD. Tibial plateau stress fracture: a complication of unicompartmental knee arthroplasty using 4 guide pins. *J Arthroplasty*. 2003;18:809–812.

5

Results of Unicompartmental Knee Arthroplasty

As noted in Chapter 1, the initial reports regarding unicompartmental knee arthroplasty (UKA) in medial compartment osteoarthritis that were published in the late 1970s were discouraging.[1,2] A few years later, Scott and Santore published more favorable results using the unicondylar prosthesis.[3] They studied 100 knees with 2- to 6-year follow-up. Three repeat operations had been performed, for an incidence of revision of roughly 1% per year at this short follow-up. The average flexion was 114 degrees, significantly better than in any contemporary reports using bicompartmental arthroplasty. When the same series was followed at 5 to 9 years (mean 7 years), seven revisions had been performed for a revision rate continuing at 1% per year.[4] The total condylar experience at that time for the same follow-up also showed a revision rate of 1% per year.[5] Armed with this information, pockets of enthusiasm for unicompartmental arthroplasty began to appear. Proponents argued that when the knee was exposed for arthroplasty and the patient fulfilled the criteria for unicompartmental replacement, it was reasonable to perform this procedure. It was conservative regarding bone resection, preserved both cruciate ligaments, yielded knees with range of motion superior to that normally achieved with total knee arthroplasty (TKA), had competitive survivorship, and was relatively easy to convert should that be required in the future (see Chapter 10).

As experience with unicompartmental arthroplasty increased, indications were expanded, numbers increased, and results could now be isolated into multiple different categories such as the "classic candidate" and "outliers," such as the anterior cruciate ligament (ACL)-deficient knee, patients with osteonecrosis, middle-aged patients, and octogenarians. These outlier categories are discussed in more detail in Chapter 9.

RESULTS IN THE "CLASSIC CANDIDATE"

UKA is an attractive and reliable option for the treatment of isolated medial or lateral compartment osteoarthritis. UKA has the advantages of improved functional outcome, higher patient satisfaction, preserved knee kinematics, faster recovery, preservation of bone, and fewer complications compared with TKA.[6–10] Similarly, UKA has longer survivorship and fewer complications than high tibial osteotomy at 10- and 15-year follow-up.[11]

Ten-year follow-up of multiple implants have consistently shown that UKA survivorship is greater than 90% where survivorship is defined as revision and radiographic signs of loosening.[12–15] National registry data shows that this is true for both cementless and cemented UKA amongst high-volume surgeons (30 or more cases per year), with 10-year survivorship of 97.5% for cementless UKA and 94.2% for cemented UKA.[16] For low- (<10 cases/year) and medium-volume (10–29 cases/year) surgeons, the 10-year implant survival rates are 86.8% and 94.3% for cementless UKA, respectively.[16] A metaanalysis of the Oxford medial unicompartmental arthroplasty including 15 studies and 8658 knees showed that the annual revision was 0.74% per 100 component years, corresponding to a 10-year survival of 93% and 15-year survival of 89%.[17] The authors additionally found that UKA outperformed TKA for patient-reported outcomes, medical complication rate, and nonrevision reoperation rate.[17] There was a higher rate of revision for UKA than TKA, usually for conversion of UKA to TKA, but UKA had a lower rate of overall nonrevision reoperation than TKA.[17]

Beyond long-term survivorship, well-selected patients undergoing UKA have excellent functional outcomes that are often better than what is reported for TKA. For example, patients undergoing UKA have better quadriceps function, gait, knee flexion, and earlier return to work than for those with TKA.[10,12,18,19]

However, despite the benefits of UKA, the long-term survival rate of UKA remains inferior to that of TKA.[12,20] Aseptic loosening, pain, infection, unequal polyethylene wear, and progression of osteoarthritis are common causes of revision.[21–24] It has been proposed that these failures and revisions may be due in part to poor patient selection, postoperative limb malalignment, and poor implant positioning.[21–24] In a study by Chatellard et al., it was shown that low implant survivorship was associated with tibial component obliquity and tibial slope that exceeded a deviation of 3 degrees and 5 degrees, respectively.[22] Other studies have similarly attributed early failures to component malpositioning and inappropriate soft tissue balancing.[24] It has been proposed that undercorrection of preoperative angular deformity can reduce the risk of overstuffing and thus minimize polyethlene wear.[12]

Taken together, well-selected patients do well after UKA and have excellent survivorship of their implants when paired with good surgical technique, failing at a rate of less than 1% per year of follow-up.

REFERENCES

1. Insall J, Walker P. Unicondylar knee replacement. *Clin Orthop Relat Res*. 1976:(120);83–85.
2. Laskin R. Unicompartmental tibiofemoral resurfacing arthroplasty. *J Bone Joint Surg Am*. 1978;60:182–185.
3. Scott RD, Santore RF. Unicondylar unicompartmental replacement for osteoarthritis of the knee. *J Bone Joint Surg Am*. 1981;63:536–544.
4. Scott RD, Cobb AG, McQueary FG, Thornhill TS. Unicompartmental knee arthroplasty. Eight- to 12-year follow-up evaluation with survivorship analysis. *Clin Orthop Relat Res*. 1992;(271):96–100.
5. Insall JN, Hood RW, Flawn LB, Sullivan DJ. The total condylar knee prosthesis in gonarthrosis. A five to nine-year follow-up of the first one hundred consecutive replacements. *J Bone Joint Surg Am*. 1983;65:619–628.
6. Flury A, Hasler J, Dimitriou D, Antoniadis A, Finsterwald M, Helmy N. Midterm clinical and radiographic outcomes of 115 consecutive patient-specific unicompartmental knee arthroplasties. *Knee*. 2019;26:889–896.
7. Bell SW, Anthony I, Jones B, MacLean A, Rowe P, Blyth M. Improved accuracy of component positioning with robotic-assisted unicompartmental knee arthroplasty. *J Bone Joint Surg Am*. 2016;98:627–635.
8. Patil S, Colwell CW, Ezzet KA, D'Lima DD. Can normal knee kinematics be restored with unicompartmental knee replacement? *J Bone Joint Surg Am*. 2005;87:332–338.
9. Morris MJ, Molli RG, Berend KR, Lombardi AV. Mortality and perioperative complications after unicompartmental knee arthroplasty. *Knee*. 2013;20:218–220.
10. Chassin EP, Mikosz RP, Andriacchi TP, Rosenberg AG. Functional analysis of cemented medial unicompartmental knee arthroplasty. *J Arthroplasty*. 1996;11:553–559.
11. Weale AE, Newman JH. Unicompartmental arthroplasty and high tibial osteotomy for osteoarthrosis of the knee. A comparative study with a 12- to 17-year follow-up period. *Clin Orthop Relat Res*. 1994;(302):134–137.
12. Berger RA, Meneghini RM, Jacobs JJ, et al. Results of unicompartmental knee arthroplasty at a minimum of ten years of follow-up. *J Bone Joint Surg Am*. 2005; 87:999–1006.
13. Murray DW, Goodfellow JW, O'Connor JJ. The Oxford medial unicompartmental arthroplasty. A ten-year survival study. *J Bone Joint Surg Br*. 1998;80:983–989.
14. Squire MW, Callaghan JJ, Goetz DD, Sullivan PM, Johnston RC. Unicompartmental knee replacement. A minimum 15 year followup study. *Clin Orthop Relat Res*. 1999;(367):61–72.
15. Svärd UC, Price AJ. Oxford medial unicompartmental knee arthroplasty. A survival analysis of an independent series. *J Bone Joint Surg Br*. 2001;83:191–194.
16. Mohammad HR, Matharu GS, Judge A, Murray DW. The effect of surgeon caseload on the relative revision rate of cemented and cementless unicompartmental knee replacements: an analysis from the National Joint Registry for England, Wales, Northern Ireland and the Isle of Man. *J Bone Joint Surg Am*. 2020;102:644–653.
17. Mohammad HR, Strickland L, Hamilton TW, Murray DW. Long-term outcomes of over 8,000 medial Oxford phase 3 unicompartmental knees-a systematic review. *Acta Orthop*. 2018;89:101–107.
18. Andriacchi TP, Galante JO, Fermier RW. The influence of total knee-replacement design on walking and stair-climbing. *J Bone Joint Surg Am*. 1982;64(9):1328–1335.
19. Kievit AJ, Kuijer PPFM, de Haan LJ, et al. Patients return to work sooner after unicompartmental knee arthroplasty than after total knee arthroplasty. *Knee Surg Sports Traumatol Arthrosc*. 2020;28:2905–2916.
20. Newman J, Pydisetty RV, Ackroyd C. Unicompartmental or total knee replacement: the 15-year results of a prospective randomised controlled trial. *J Bone Joint Surg Br*. 2009;91:52–57.
21. Hernigou P, Deschamps G. Alignment influences wear in the knee after medial unicompartmental arthroplasty. *Clin Orthop Relat Res*. 2004;(423):161–165. doi:10.1097/01.blo.0000128285.90459.12.

22. Chatellard R, Sauleau V, Colmar M, Robert H, Raynaud G, Brilhault J. Medial unicompartmental knee arthroplasty: does tibial component position influence clinical outcomes and arthroplasty survival? *Orthop Traumatol Surg Res*. 2013;99:S219–S225.
23. Pearle AD, van der List JP, Lee L, Coon TM, Borus TA, Roche MW. Survivorship and patient satisfaction of robotic-assisted medial unicompartmental knee arthroplasty at a minimum two-year follow-up. *Knee*. 2017;24:419–428.
24. Epinette JA, Brunschweiler B, Mertl P, Mole D, Cazenave A. Unicompartmental knee arthroplasty modes of failure: wear is not the main reason for failure: a multicentre study of 418 failed knees. *Orthop Traumatol Surg Res*. 2012;98: S124–S130.

6

Surgical Technique of Medial Fixed-Bearing Unicompartmental Knee Arthroplasty

INTRAOPERATIVE CONFIRMATION OF PATIENT CANDIDACY

Even if a unicompartmental knee arthroplasty (UKA) is planned for a patient based on preoperative radiographs and physical examination, the surgeon must confirm at arthrotomy that the patient is an appropriate candidate. Both cruciate ligaments should be intact, although a deficient anterior cruciate ligament (ACL) is occasionally acceptable for fixed-bearing UKA if certain criteria are fulfilled (see Chapter 9).

Secondly, there should be no sign of significant mediolateral tibiofemoral subluxation. Evidence of this form of instability is the finding of a so-called "kissing lesion" on the medial aspect of the lateral femoral condyle. This lesion usually consists of a divot secondary to impingement of the lateral tibial spine on the lateral condyle along with an accompanying osteophyte. Although this lesion can usually be seen on a preoperative radiograph, especially a posteroanterior (PA) flexed view, intraoperative assessment is especially important to determine its significance. A large lesion may indicate that medial–lateral stability cannot be restored to the knee by a UKA, whereas a smaller lesion merely requires debridement of the accompanying impinging osteophyte (Fig. 6.1).

Changes no greater than grade I should be present in the opposite compartment.[1] The patellofemoral compartment can have up to grade III changes, but the presence of eburnated bone in the lateral patellar facet is probably a contraindication to the procedure.[2] Significant inflammatory synovitis is an absolute contraindication especially in the presence of crystalline disease in the form of gout or pseudogout. If there is no synovial inflammation at surgery and no history of inflammatory episodes in the past, many surgeons do not consider crystalline disease a contraindication to UKA.

GENERIC SURGICAL TECHNIQUE

The technique that follows is as generic as possible regarding fixed-bearing UKA. Each prosthetic design will have individualized features in alignment, cutting jigs, and modes of prosthetic fixation such as lugs or fins. Chapter 7 covers mobile-bearing technique.

Basic Principles

A significant advantage of UKA is its potentially conservative nature. It preserves both cruciate ligaments, the opposite compartment, and the patellofemoral articulation. If the prosthetic design and surgical technique remain conservative, bone is also preserved in the compartment being resurfaced. The goal should be to prepare a unicompartmental replacement in such a way that no augmentation methods will be necessary at the time of any future revision. The only possible deficiency occurring at revision of a medial UKA should be on the tibial side resulting from subsidence of the tibial component. Fortunately, osteolysis compromising bone stock is extremely rare in UKA.

The following are the basic principles for medial unicompartmental arthroplasty:

- Conservative tibia-first resection
- Assessment of the resultant flexion and extension gaps
- Equalization of the gaps
- Distal femoral resection in the proper alignment and amount
- Sizing the femur and aligning it relative to the tibia in 90 degrees of flexion
- Completion of the femoral preparation
- Sizing, orienting, and completing tibial preparation
- Confirmation of limb alignment and component orientation with trial components
- Implantation of real components

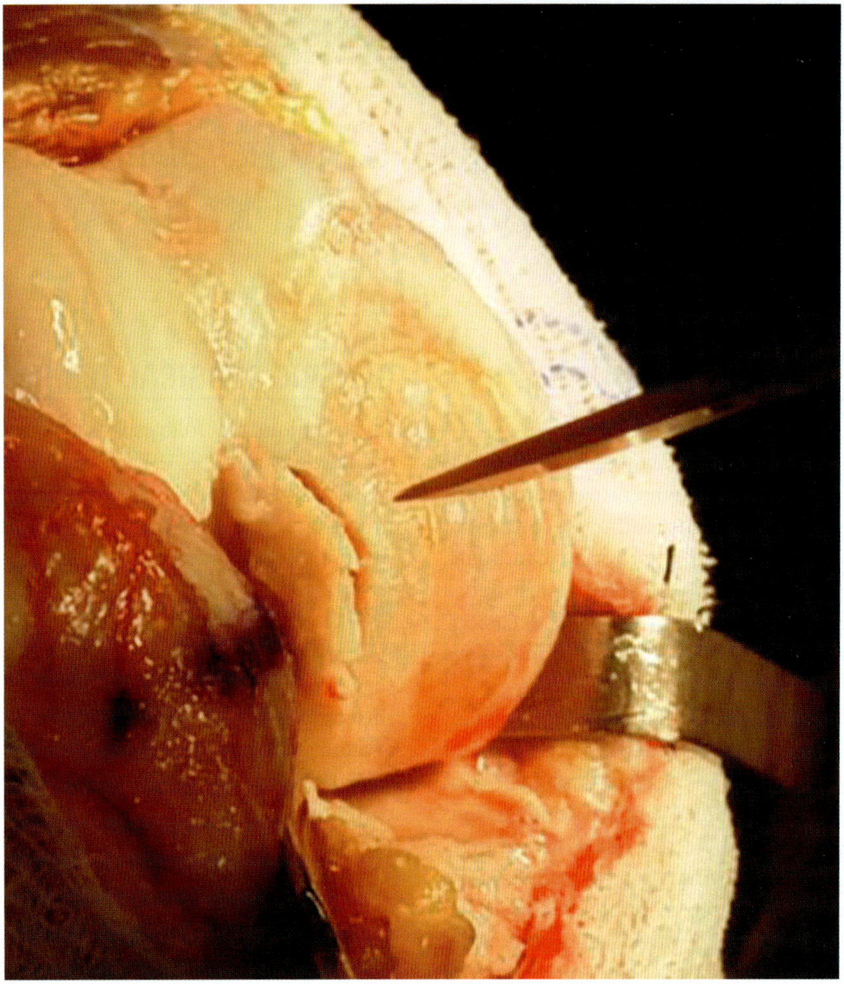

Fig. 6.1 Intercondylar femoral osteophytes should be removed to define the anatomy of the medial femoral condyle, relieve any intercondylar impingement, and provide a pathway for a reciprocal saw utilized to complete the tibial resection.

Preoperative Planning

To accomplish a conservative tibia-first preparation, the preoperative anteroposterior radiographs should be used to plan the level of the resection. A conservative resection line is drawn on the radiograph at 90 degrees to the long axis of the tibia (Fig. 6.2). The level of this resection is determined on the lateral side 8 to 10 mm below the joint line. The level of the initial tibial resection should be no lower than this line, whether it is for a medial or a lateral compartment arthroplasty. For medial compartment replacement, the resection begins where this line intersects with the most peripheral aspect of the plateau. For most knees, this will be between 0 and 2 mm of peripheral tibial resection. This amount of resection makes sense, because the authors' experience has shown that for every millimeter of elevation of the joint line from the periphery of the plateau, approximately 1 degree of correction is obtained. Therefore, if the peripheral resection is 0 and a 7-mm tibial component is used, approximately 7 degrees of correction will be achieved. This would convert a typical UKA candidate in 3 degrees of anatomic varus to 4 degrees of anatomic valgus (Fig. 6.3).

Operative Exposure

Traditionally, UKA of the medial side was performed by a standard total knee exposure using a median parapatellar

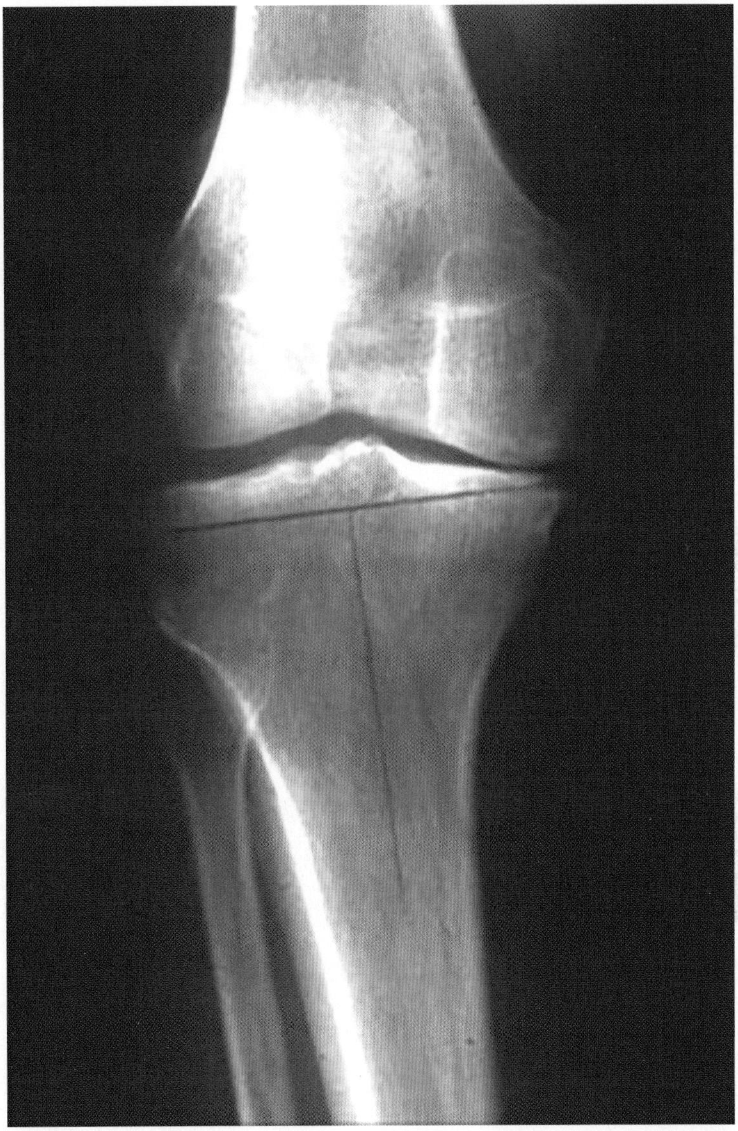

Fig. 6.2 Preoperative planning for a medial unicompartmental knee arthroplasty involves drawing a conservative resection for total knee arthroplasty with a line 90 degrees to the long axis of the tibia that is 8 to 10 mm below the lateral joint line. The amount of peripheral medial tibial resection is usually 0 to 2 mm, as shown on this radiograph.

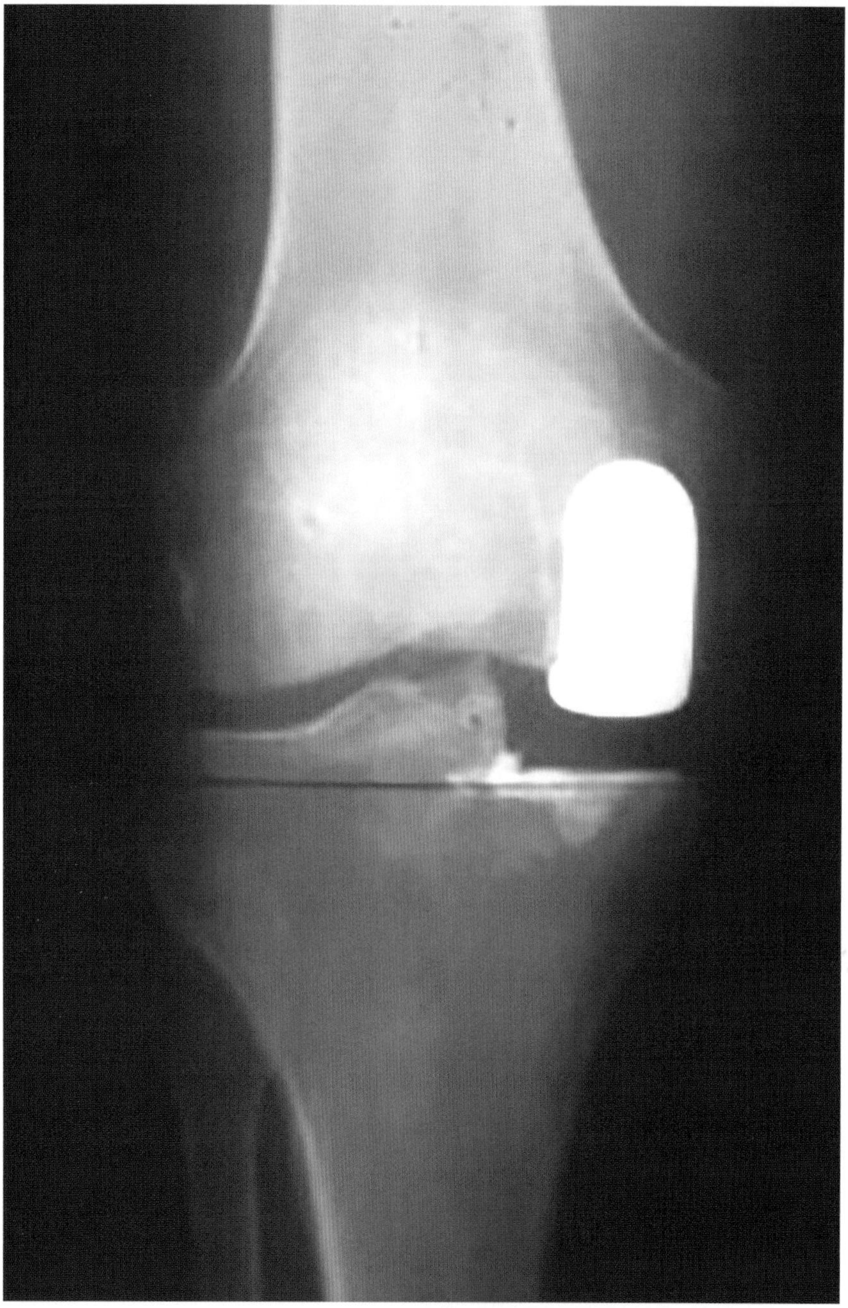

Fig. 6.3 A postoperative radiograph showing how a tibial resection of zero from the peripheral medial plateau combined with a 7-mm tibial component corrects the preoperative anatomic alignment.

arthrotomy with complete eversion of the patella. Care would be taken not to derange the anterior horn of the lateral meniscus. This exposure gave the surgeon the opportunity to completely explore the knee and make an intraoperative decision about whether the patient was a candidate for UKA.

Minimally invasive unicompartmental surgery is now the standard.[3] The shorter incisions permit a shorter hospital stay (possibly even outpatient surgery) and a faster recovery due to less disruption of the quadriceps. If a surgeon prefers a somewhat larger arthrotomy, however, rapid recovery is possible if the patella is subluxed laterally rather than everted.

A shorter than normal skin incision typically used for a TKA is appropriate. It can be approximately 8 to 10 cm in length. The arthrotomy begins just above the superior pole of the patella. It ends distally at the midportion of the tibial tubercle. Adequate inspection of the joint can usually be accomplished by flexing the knee 30 to 40 degrees and manually subluxating the patella. Digital palpation of the patella allows for the detection of eburnated bone on its surface. A retractor such as a bent Hohmann is anchored in the intercondylar notch and allows maintenance of the lateral subluxation of the patella during the procedure (Fig. 6.4). For lateral compartment replacement exposure, see Chapter 8.

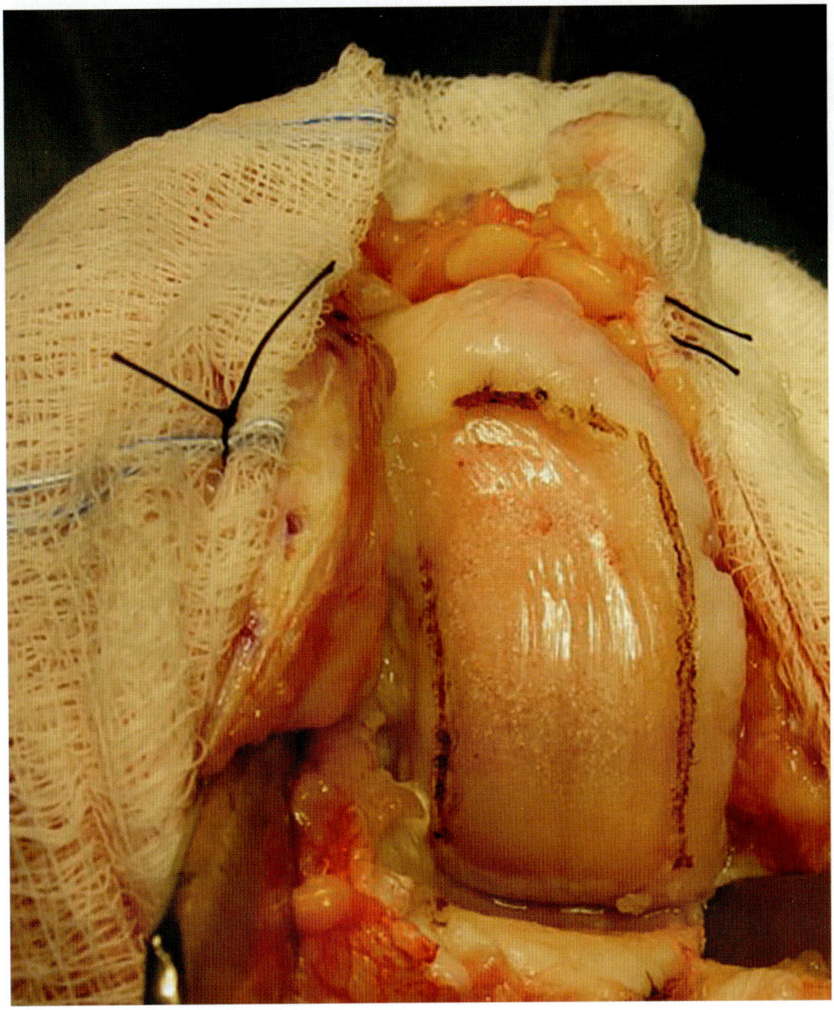

Fig. 6.4 Excellent exposure of the medial compartment can be achieved through a short medial arthrotomy with subluxation of the patella using a bent Hohmann retractor.

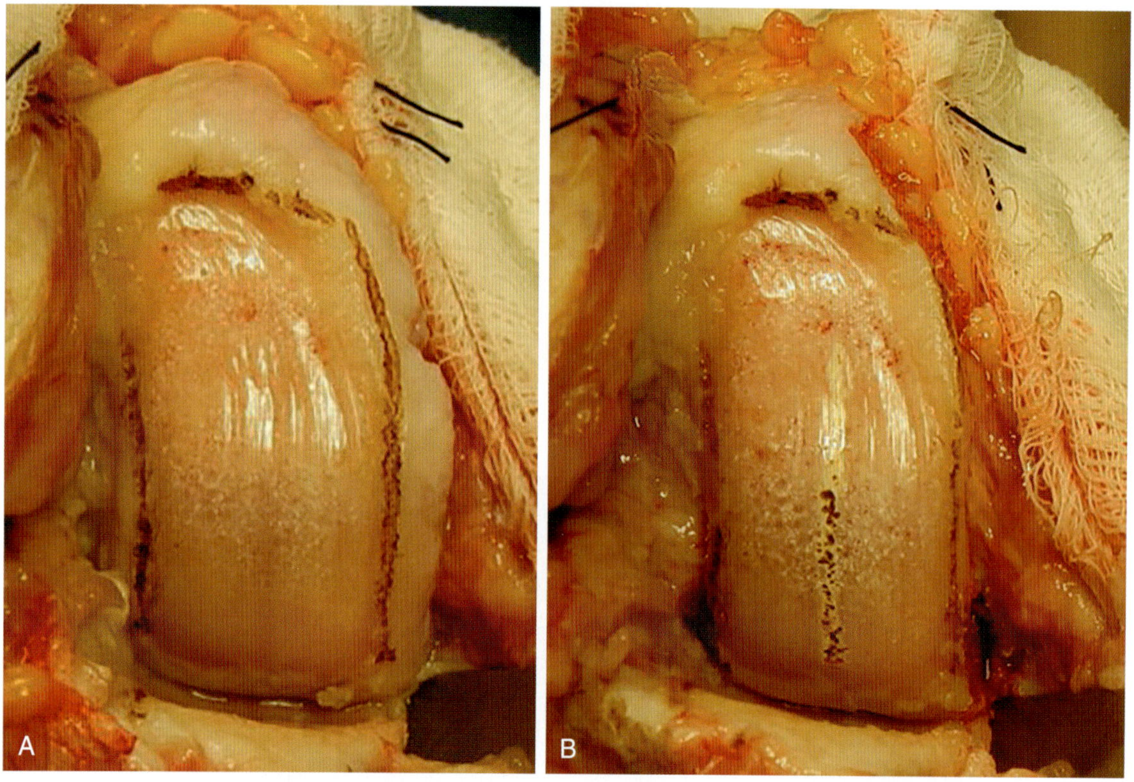

Fig. 6.5 (A) In this isolated view of the medial femoral condyle, the "tide-mark" junction between the trochlear cartilage and the eburnated condylar bone is easily defined along with the intercondylar and medial femoral osteophytes. (B) The osteophytes have been removed to precisely define the femoral condylar anatomy.

Other Elements of Medial Exposure

Before execution of the bony resections, the anatomy should be defined. This includes outlining the medial and intercondylar femoral osteophytes and the so-called "tide-mark" which is the most anterior aspect of the medial articulation (Fig. 6.5A). Medial and intercondylar osteophytes are then removed to define the true mediolateral dimension of the condyle (Fig. 6.5B). Removal of intercondylar osteophytes also relieves any potential impingement between them and the tibial spine and provides a pathway for the resection that will take place along the spine. Removal of medial osteophytes also releases the medial collateral ligament (MCL) and allows passive correction of the deformity (Fig. 6.6).

The chondro-osseous wear pattern on the femoral condyle femur can be defined with a marking pen or electrocautery. This gives an initial guide to the proper rotatory alignment of the femoral component (Fig. 6.7). Final rotational alignment of both the femoral and tibial component is established as the bone preparation proceeds and trials are placed.

Preparation of the Tibia

The description given here applies to the technique for an "on-lay" type of tibial component. The same general principles of preparation apply for an "in-lay" technique. Measures should be taken to protect the MCL from injury. After the anterior third of the medial meniscus is removed, an entry point can be defined between the deep MCL and the proximal tibial plateau. At this level, a curved 1-cm osteotome is inserted tangential to the plateau, with half its surface above and the other half below the level of the plateau. It is then tapped with a mallet along the border of the plateau until it reaches the level of the semimembranosus bursa. This creates a pathway for insertion of a retractor that will protect the MCL during tibial preparation.

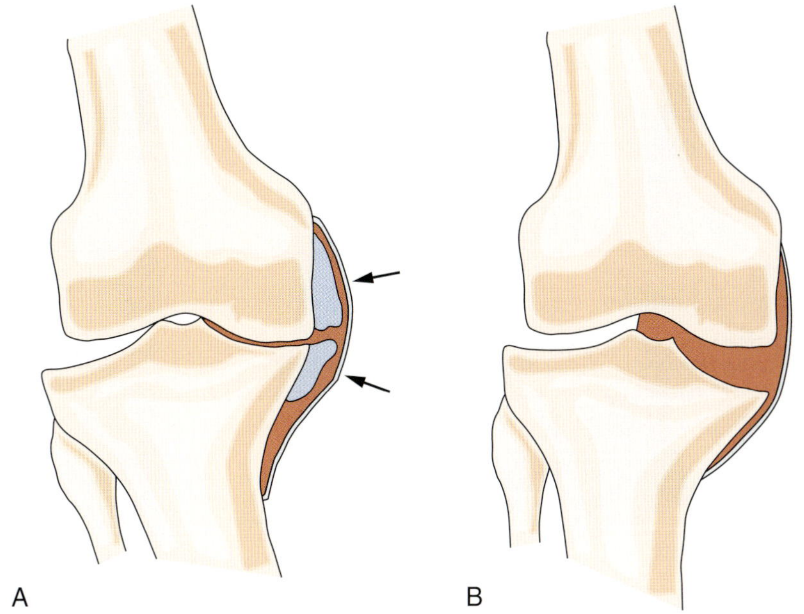

Fig. 6.6 (A) The typical medial femoral and tibial osteophytes seen in varus osteoarthritis are shown diagrammatically tenting up the medial collateral ligament. (B) After removal of the osteophytes, the resultant laxity allows passive correction of the varus deformity.

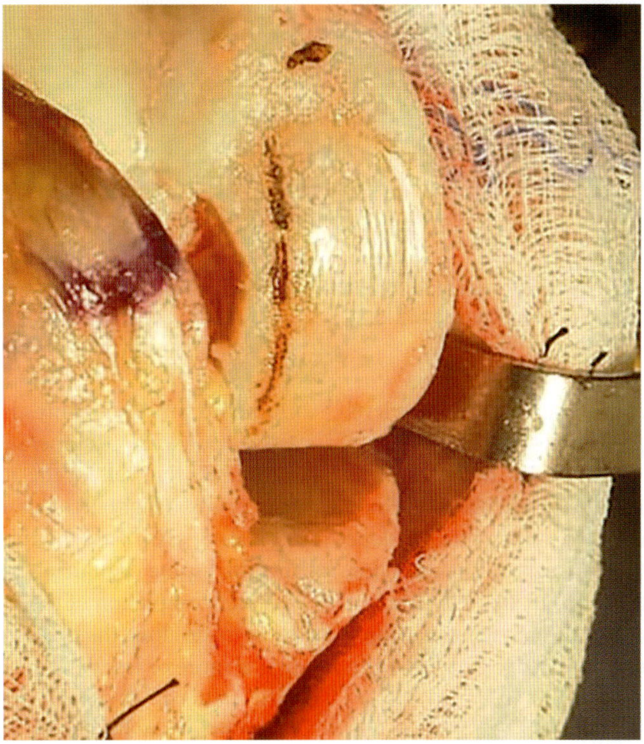

Fig. 6.7 The chondro-osseous wear pattern of the femoral surface has been marked with electrocautery.

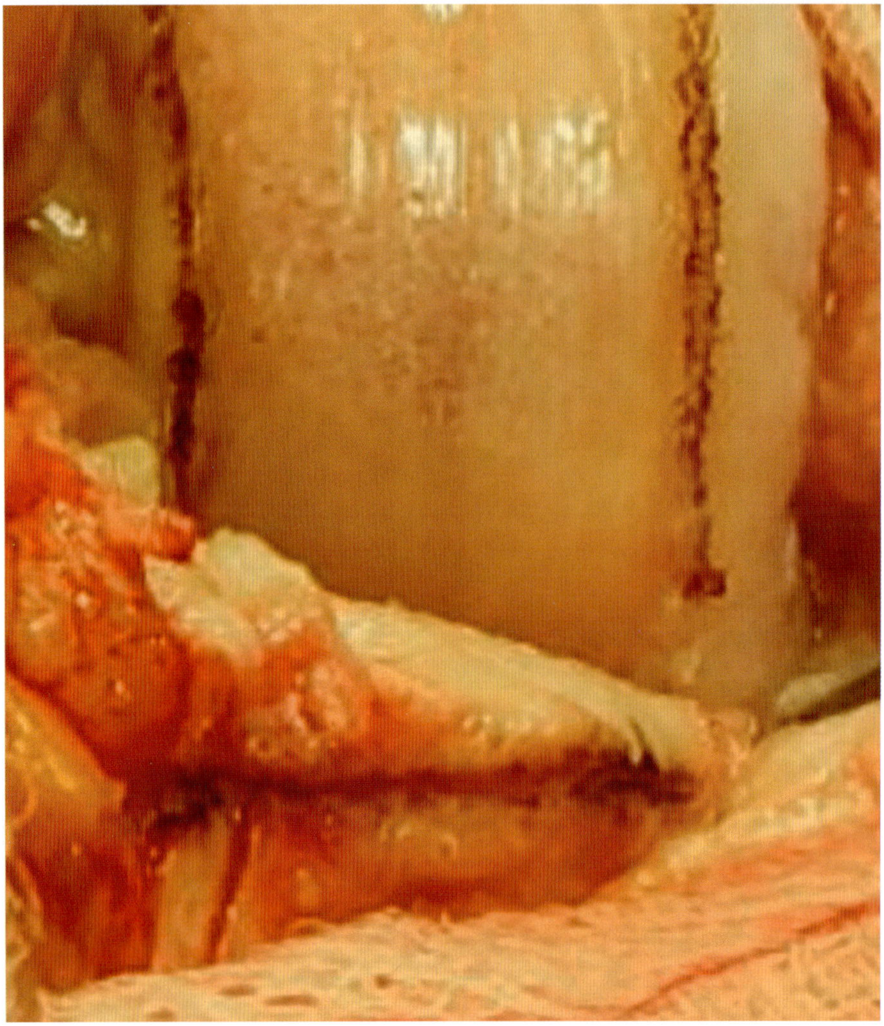

Fig. 6.8 A line for a conservative initial tibial resection has been marked on the tibial bone to correlate with the preoperative templated resection (see Fig. 6.2).

An external tibial alignment jig is applied, with the level of resection based on the preoperative templating for a conservative cut (Fig. 6.8; see also Fig. 6.2). The varus/valgus alignment should be more or less perpendicular to the long axis of the tibia and the amount of initial posterior slope applied should be between 3 and 5 degrees. The exception to this amount of slope is for a qualifying ACL-deficient knee (see Chapter 9) and for lateral compartment arthroplasties in which posterior slope is limited to between 0 and 3 degrees (see Chapter 8).

If the alignment jig is to be stabilized by a fixation pin, it is recommended that only one inboard pin be used. Outboard pins that come close to the medial cortex are associated with postoperative stress fractures, as are techniques that call for the application of multiple stabilizing pins[4] (Fig. 6.9). It is important to use a narrow oscillating saw blade for this cut to avoid undercutting the tibial spine or injuring medial soft tissues (Fig. 6.10).

After completion of the horizontal bone cut, a vertical cut is made along the tibial spine with a reciprocating saw that is more or less parallel to the tibial chondro-osseous wear pattern. As noted previously, a medial femoral osteophyte may have to be removed to create a pathway for the saw. The lateral placement of this cut is, in general,

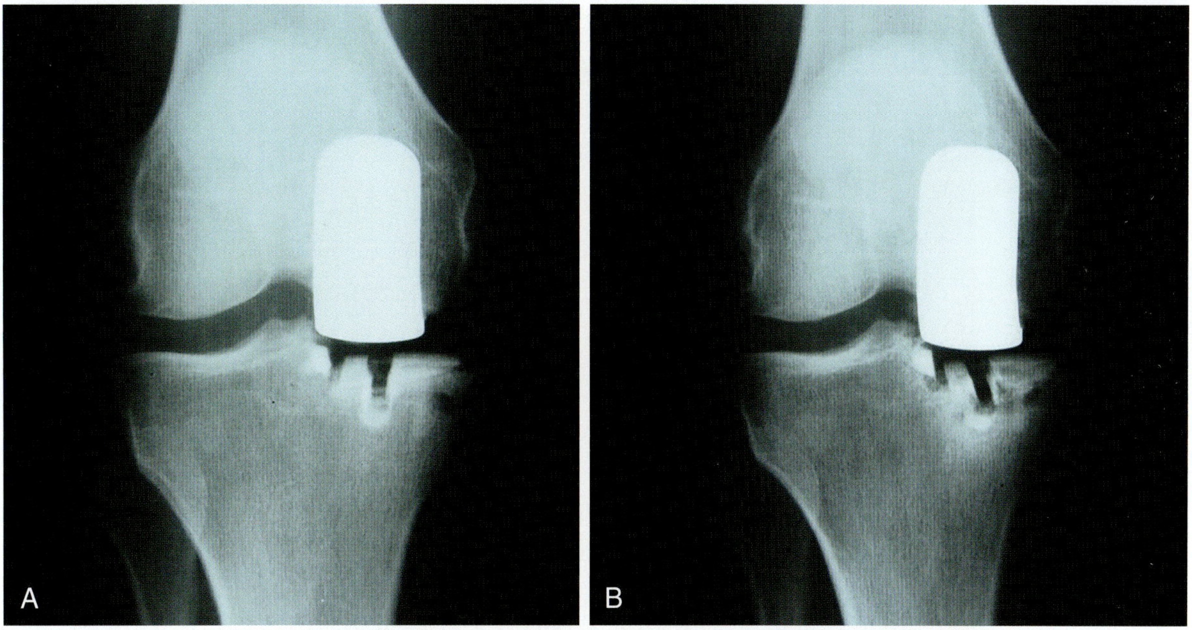

Fig. 6.9 (A) A peripheral pin hole placed for an alignment jig created a stress riser. (B) In this case, a postoperative stress fracture occurred through that pin hole.

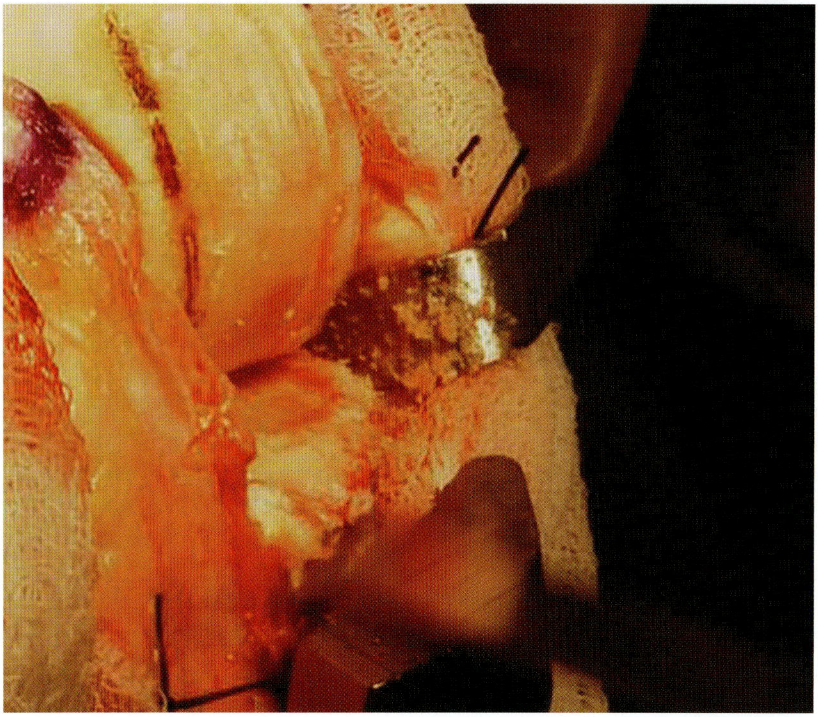

Fig. 6.10 This intraoperative photograph shows a medial retractor protecting the soft tissues during the tibial resection.

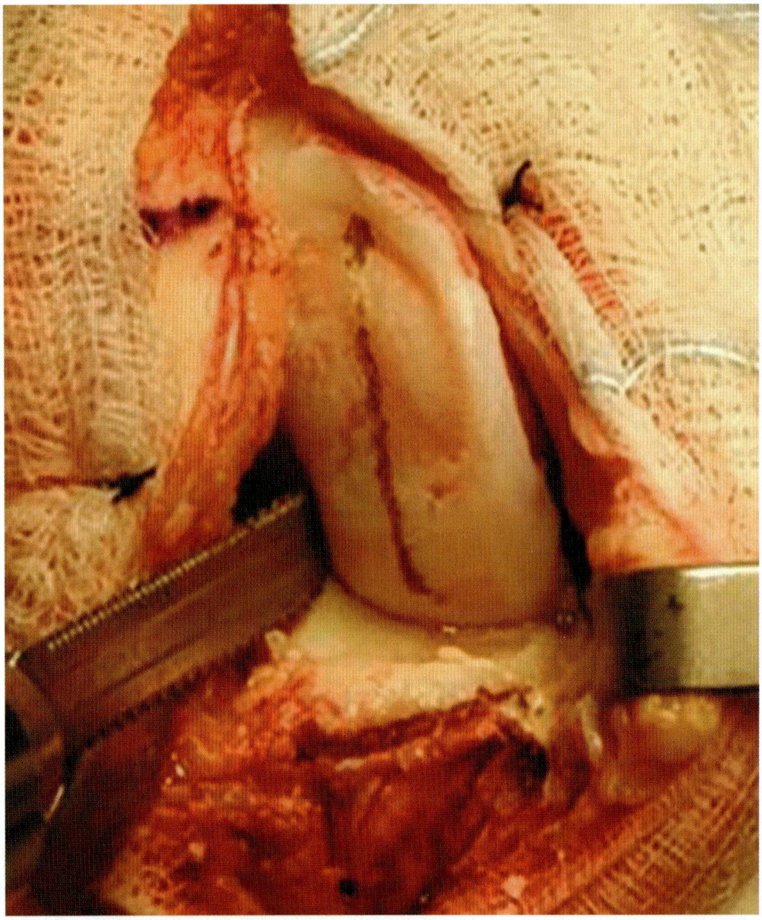

Fig. 6.11 The tibial resection is completed with a vertical cut halfway up the slope of the medial tibial spine.

halfway up the slope of the medial tibial spine (Fig. 6.11). The resected tibial bone is easier to remove with the knee in extension than in flexion because cartilage usually remains posteriorly on both femur and tibia in isolated medial osteoarthritis. The resected bone can be grasped with a Kocher clamp while the knee is in flexion and then pulled free when the knee is extended. The resected piece will usually show a wear pattern that is anterior and medial (Fig. 6.12).

With the knee in extension, the thinnest tibial trial is slid into the space created by the tibial resection (Fig. 6.13). If this tibial thickness is correct, the knee should come to full extension and the anatomic alignment should lie between 2 and 5 degrees of valgus. The knee should be stable to valgus stress. It is permissible for the medial side to spring open 1 or 2 mm with the valgus stress but not remain open by this amount when the stress is released. If the alignment is undercorrected or the medial side is lax, a thicker trial insert is necessary. Alternatively, the distal femoral resection can be less than anatomic to allow tightening of the extension gap. Deciding between these alternatives depends on the corresponding flexion gap. For example, if both extension gap and flexion gap are loose, a thicker tibial insert is appropriate. If the extension gap is loose but the flexion gap is appropriate, diminished distal femoral resection is recommended.

Once the extension gap has been established, the same thickness of trial tibial component is tested in flexion. The medial retractor should be relaxed during this test or it might create a false sense of tightness. Under ideal circumstances, the appropriate trial for extension stability slides in easily under the posterior condyle with the knee

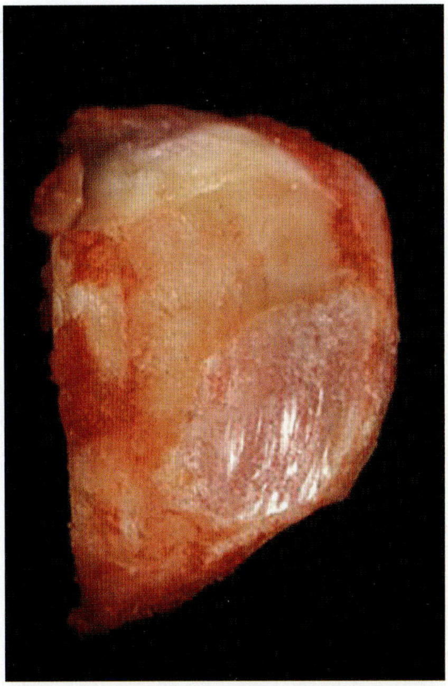

Fig. 6.12 This tibial resection demonstrates the classic anteromedial wear pattern seen in medial osteoarthritis.

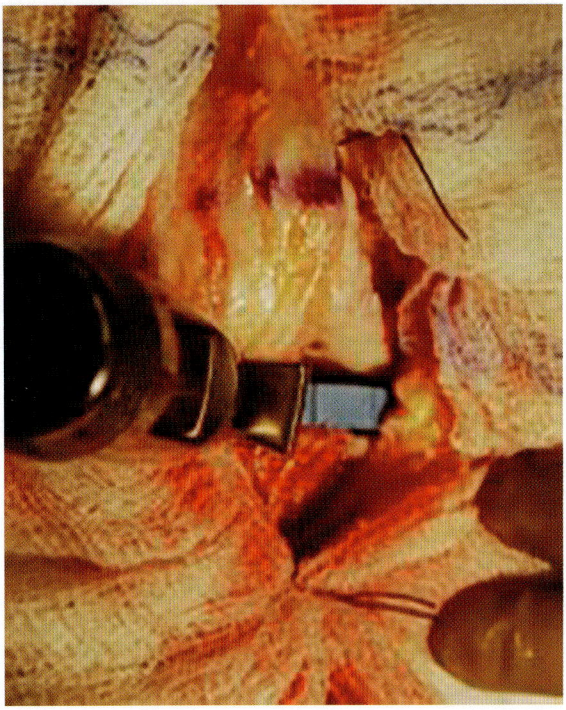

Fig. 6.13 The thinnest tibial trial has been inserted and the knee brought to full extension to assess its effect on alignment and stability. The tibial thickness that allows full extension (without hyperextension) while restoring alignment and stability, establishes the extension gap.

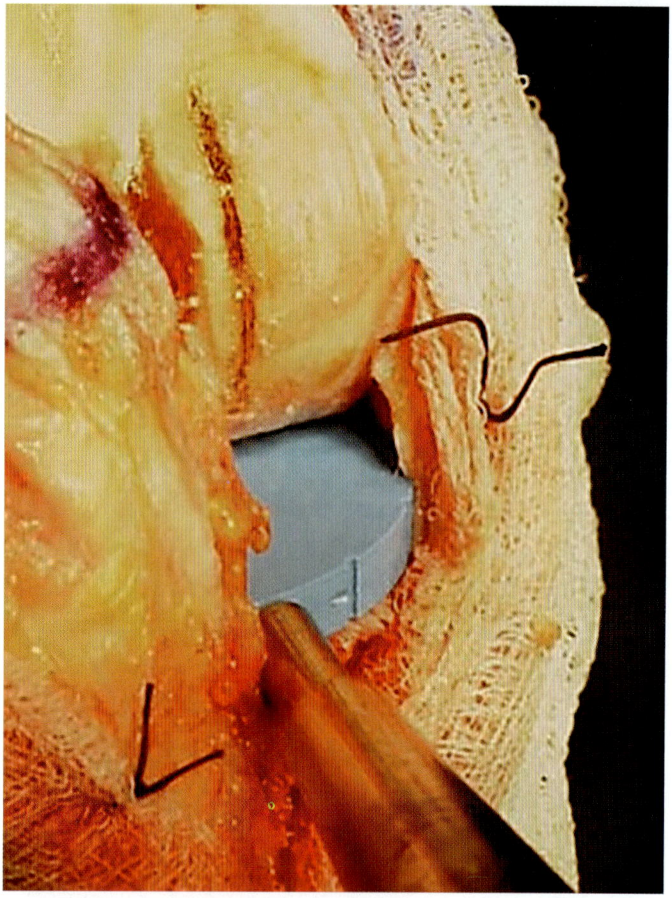

Fig. 6.14 The same thickness of tibial trial chosen in extension is now assessed in 90 degrees of knee flexion. Any medial retractor should be removed or relaxed (see text).

flexed 90 degrees (Fig. 6.14). Erring toward the slightly lax side in flexion is better than erring toward the slightly tight side. To relieve flexion tightness for any given tibial thickness, the trial insert is pushed into the flexion space until it engages the posterior condyle (Fig. 6.15). A line is then drawn parallel to the top of the insert to show the angle of resection necessary to increase the flexion space. This resection can be performed with the narrow oscillating saw. It usually amounts to 1 or 2 mm and often only involves removal of residual posterior condylar cartilage.

If both the flexion and extension spaces are too tight, a little more of the tibia may be resected but the surgeon must remain as conservative as possible on the tibial side. If the spacing is fine in flexion but tight in extension, the surgeon can resect a little more than the anatomic amount of distal femur that corresponds with the thickness of the femoral component. If the gap is fine in flexion but loose in extension, the distal femoral condyle is underresected.

Distal Femoral Resection

Distal femoral resection angle and amount can be guided by intramedullary or extramedullary alignment. The advantage of intramedullary alignment is its accuracy; its disadvantage is its invasiveness. Regardless of the technique, the goal is to remove an amount of bone equivalent to the thickness of the metal femoral component to attempt to restore the femoral joint line. The ideal angle of distal femoral resection is approximately 5 degrees of valgus. The forgiveness of varying from this angle depends on the congruency of the femorotibial articulation in the coronal plane. For example, a round-on-round

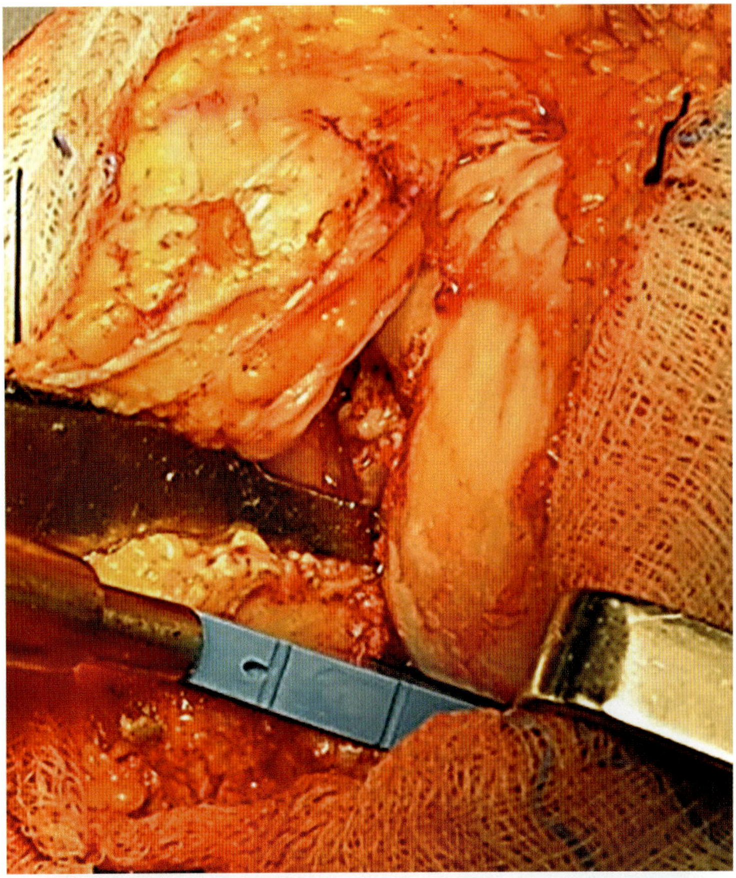

Fig. 6.15 If the appropriate tibial trial established in extension is too tight in 90 degrees of knee flexion, it is pushed up against the posterior condyle to determine the amount of residual cartilage to be removed to equalize the gaps. The amount of resection needed is usually only 1 or 2 mm and often involves removing only residual condylar cartilage (see text).

articulation as in a mobile-bearing articulation forgives any variation (see Chapter 7). A flat-on-flat articulation demands complete accuracy in the coronal alignment to avoid any edge-loading of the articulation (Fig. 6.16). Most fixed-bearing articulations are a variation of round-on-flat with the amount of forgiveness and the amount of contact area depending on the difference in the radius of curvature between one articulation and the other.

Intramedullary Femoral Alignment Technique

The medullary canal is entered similarly to that in the technique for TKA. The entry hole is approximately 1 cm above the origin of the posterior cruciate ligament (PCL) in the intercondylar notch and is usually prejudiced several millimeters to the medial side. In minimally invasive techniques, the intramedullary rod can serve to retract the patella. In most cases, the angle of distal femoral resection is set for 5 degrees of valgus.

Extramedullary Femoral Alignment Technique

In this technique, the varus/valgus alignment of the femoral component is keyed off its relationship with the previously performed tibial resection. The guide has a rectangular spacer block attached to it that is equivalent to the thickness of the tibial component selected to stabilize the knee in extension. The guide is inserted with the knee flexed between 5 and 15 degrees, depending on the amount of posterior slope applied to the tibial resection. Hyperextension of the knee while pinning the guide should be avoided because this will

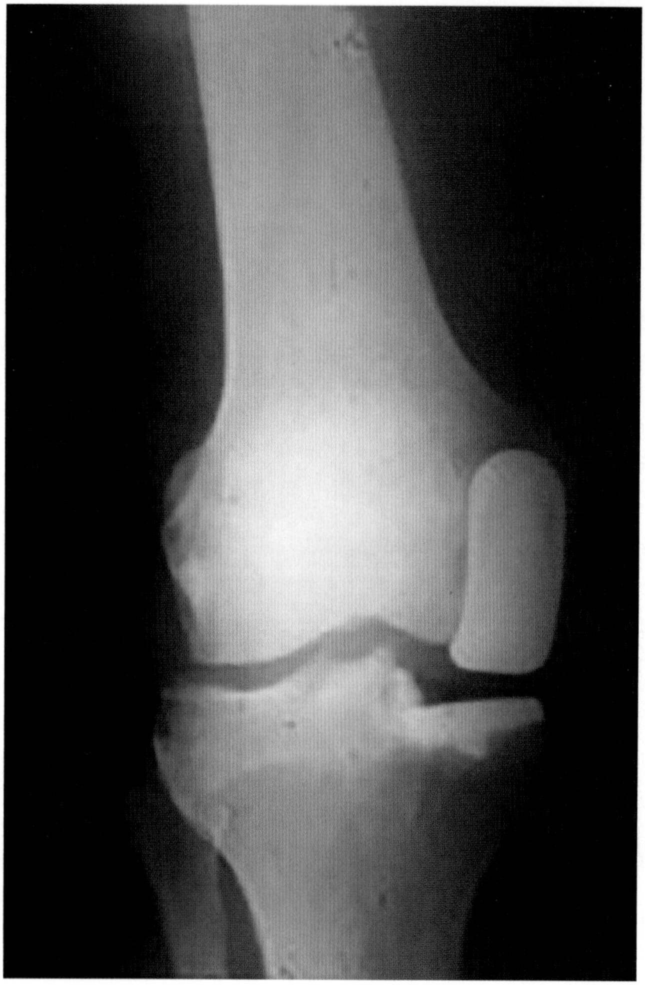

Fig. 6.16 A radiograph showing coronal misalignment between the femoral and tibial components involving a flat-on-flat articulation. This resulted in edge-loading and likely accelerated wear.

impart an extension angle to the resection with resultant extension of the femoral component (Fig. 6.17). The guide is pinned to the femur with at least two fixation pins to create stability. A cutting slot in the guide will resect the proper amount of distal condyle to restore the femoral joint line with the femoral component.

In many systems, an adaptor block can be slid onto the femoral pins to adjust the amount of resection 2 mm proximally or distally depending on the need to either increase or decrease the extension gap (Fig. 6.18).

Some systems recommend cutting the distal femur with the knee in extension. In these cases, it is difficult to visualize the progression of the cut. It may be safer to resect the distal femur with the knee in some flexion if the system permits.

Sizing of the Femur

In most UKA systems, any size of femur can be articulated with any size of tibia. For this reason, they are sized independently. The size is determined by the anteroposterior femoral dimension. For medial replacements, it is best to use the largest possible size that does not protrude anteriorly and cause patellar impingement during flexion. The rationale is that the larger size will better cap the femoral bone, providing more surface area for fixation and minimizing the chance for femoral component subsidence

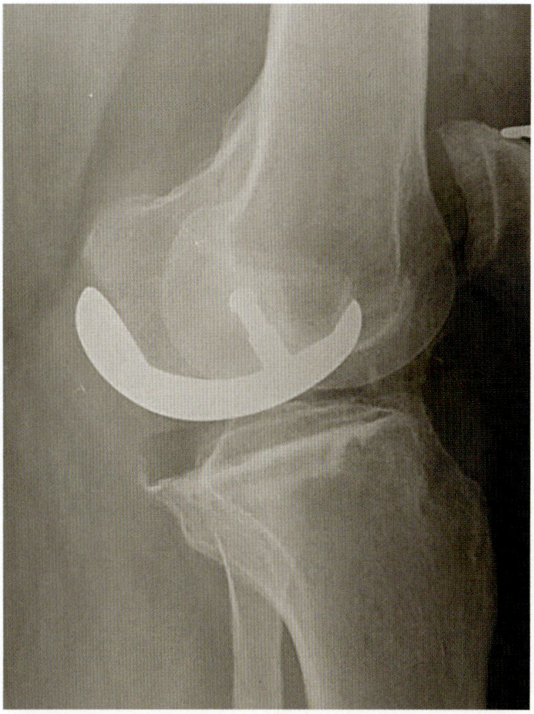

Fig. 6.17 A lateral postoperative radiograph showing hyperextension of the femoral component that occurred when the femoral resection was linked to a tibial resection performed with excessive posterior tibial slope.

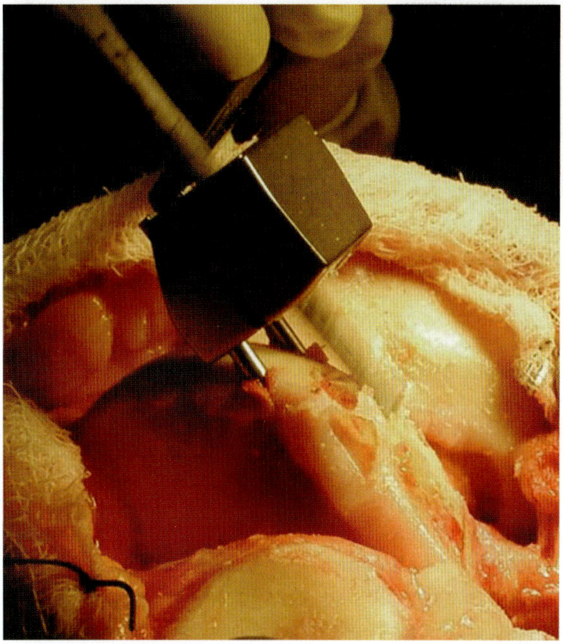

Fig. 6.18 An adapter block is available in many systems to allow for sequentially increased or decreased distal femoral resection depending on the need to increase or decrease the extension gap.

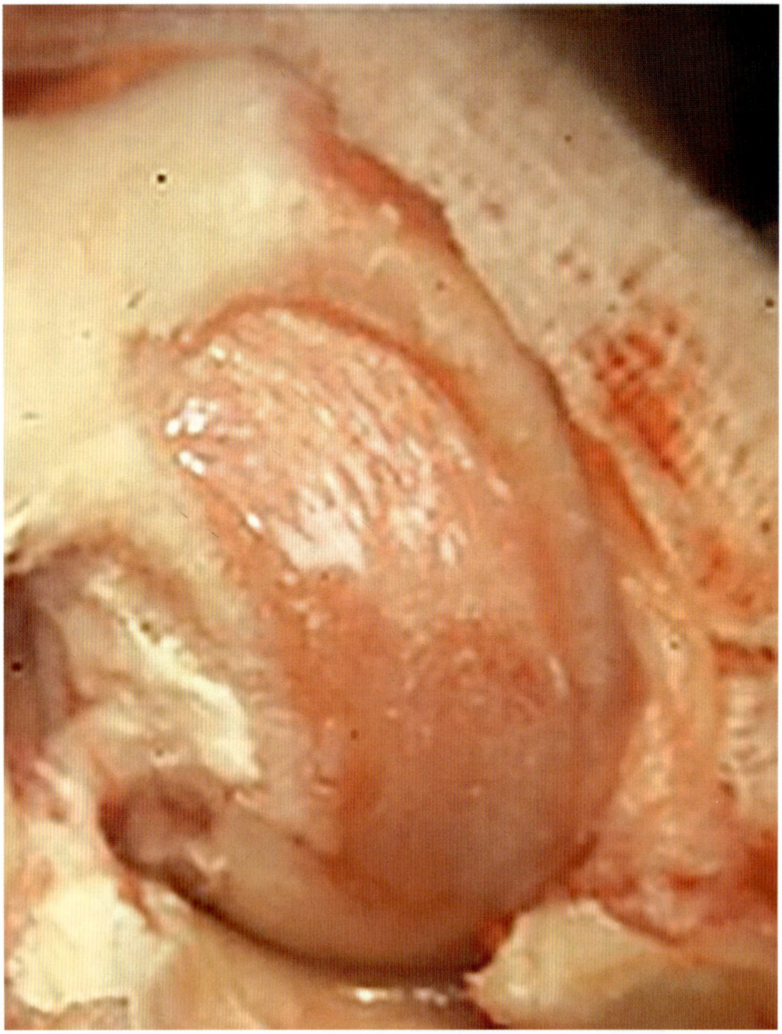

Fig. 6.19 The anatomic landmark for placement of the leading edge of the femoral component is often obvious, as shown in this intraoperative photograph.

or loosening. The anatomic landmark for the leading edge of the femoral component is sometimes obvious as the junction between intact trochlear cartilage and eburnated bone on the distal femoral condyle (Fig. 6.19).

If unclear, this landmark can be determined by placing a mark at the estimated spot and then bringing the knee to full extension to confirm metal-to-plastic contact is adequate between the femoral and tibial components with the leg in this position. Virtually all sizing jigs will key off the posterior condyle, with the anterior aspect of the guide mimicking the leading edge of the actual femoral component.

Rotational Alignment of the Femoral Component

The patient's chondro-osseous wear pattern usually suggests the appropriate rotational alignment of the femoral component (see Fig. 6.7). Another guide to rotation is to choose an alignment that is perpendicular to the varus/valgus alignment of the tibial component when the knee is flexed to 90 degrees. Choosing this alignment gives maximum congruency between the articulating surfaces in flexion. As in extension, the forgiveness of rotational discrepancies depends on the congruency of the articulating surfaces. Similar to distal alignment, a flat-on-flat articulation is very unforgiving,

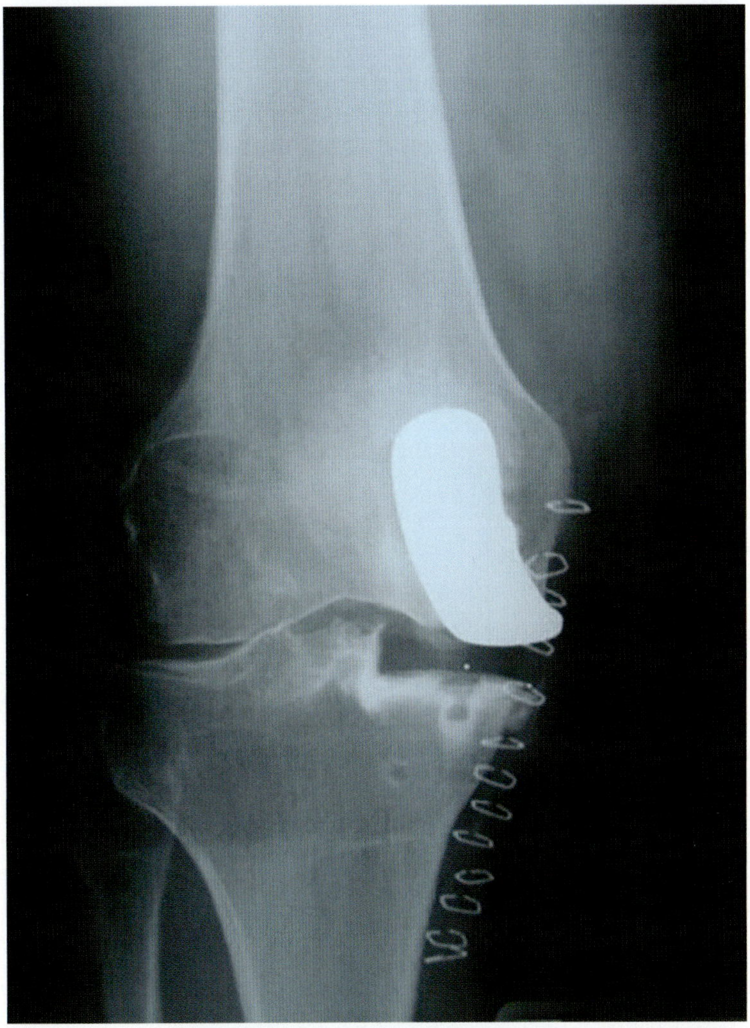

Fig. 6.20 A postoperative radiograph showing the consequence of a femoral component placed in too much internal rotation. In extension, its leading edge is tracking on the medial edge of the tibial polyethylene.

whereas a round-on-round articulation is completely forgiving. Most systems are a variation of round-on-flat with the forgiveness again dependent on the difference in radius of curvature between one articulation and the other.

Another critical aspect of femoral component rotation is its effect on the tracking of the components in full extension. The tibial wear pattern of most varus knees undergoing unicompartmental replacement is anterior and peripheral[5] (see Fig. 6.12). If the femoral component is placed in internal rotation, its leading edge will ride on the peripheral aspect of the tibial component in extension, possibly promoting premature wear and loosening (Fig. 6.20). For this reason, the surgeon should usually err toward slight external rotation of the femoral component to bring the leading edge of the femur more lateral in extension.

Mediolateral Positioning of the Femoral Component

As mentioned earlier, the usual wear pattern in early osteoarthritis in the varus knee is peripheral as well as anterior. To avoid adverse effects on the polyethylene resulting from a return to this wear pattern,[6] the femoral component should be centered on the condyle or even shifted slightly laterally. The appropriate amount of shift is determined by checking mediolateral congruency between the femoral and tibial components in full extension before making any fixation holes or slots.

Final Preparation of the Femur

Now that the proper size, rotation, and mediolateral positioning of the femoral component have been determined, the femoral resection can be completed. In most systems, this involves a posterior condylar resection, a posterior chamfer resection, and a partial anterior chamfer resection. In other techniques, a burr is used to prepare a bed for the component and angle-guided resections are not appropriate. Robotic preparation of both the femoral and tibial bone beds is an evolving technique (see Chapter 11). In all cases, a recess must be created for the leading edge of the femoral component to prevent patellar impingement (Fig. 6.21).

The trial femur is now slid into place on top of the prepared femoral bed. Some systems provide a shim to pressurize the posterior condyle up against the posterior condylar resection. It is important that a good fit be

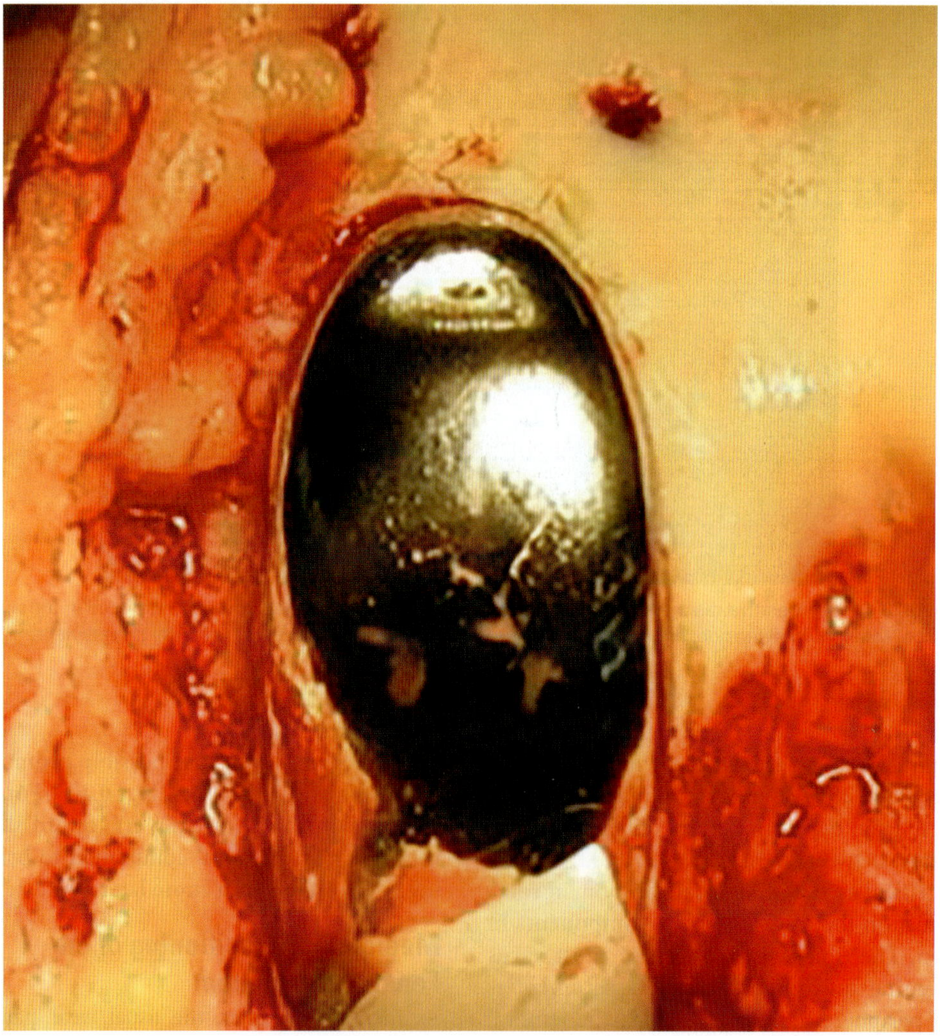

Fig. 6.21 An intraoperative photograph showing proper recession of the leading edge of the femoral component into the trochlear cartilage to minimize any chance of patellar impingement in high knee flexion.

obtained in this section of the prosthesis to resist forces that may promote femoral component loosening. In some systems, the lug fixation is parallel to the posterior condylar resection so that the component is slid into place without the potential to pressurize the cement. In other systems, femoral lugs are angled in such a way that the posterior condyle is compressed as the component is fully seated (Fig. 6.22). In systems in which the fixation lug is parallel to the posterior condyle, it may be helpful to angle the drill for the lug hole in a slightly anterior direction (Fig. 6.23).

This angling will promote slight flexion of the femoral component and compress the posterior condyle. The drill should never be angled posteriorly because this would drive the femoral component into extension and lift the metallic femoral condyle away from the bone.

Once the femur is fully prepared and the trial fully seated, it is helpful to take a curved, 6-mm wide osteotome

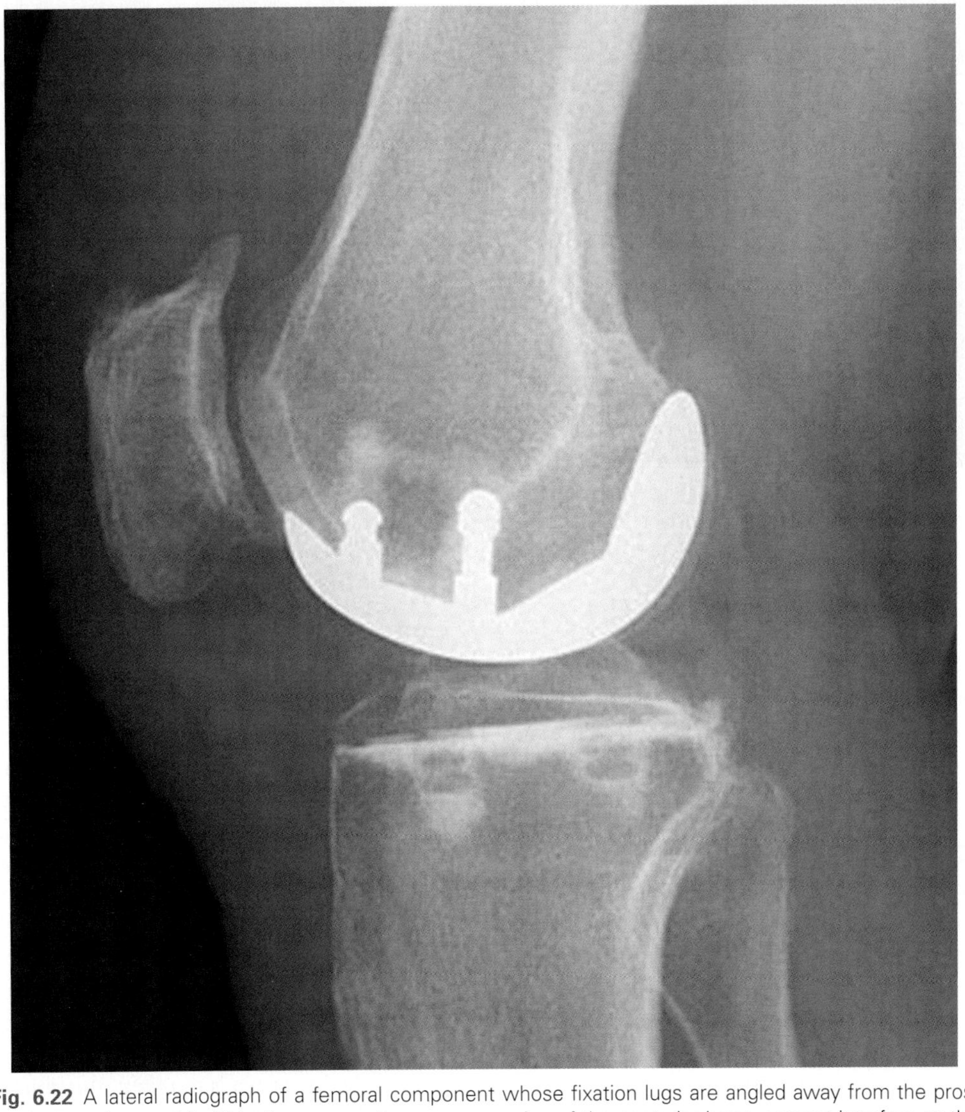

Fig. 6.22 A lateral radiograph of a femoral component whose fixation lugs are angled away from the prosthetic posterior condyle. This divergence allows compression of the posterior bone–cement interface as the component is inserted.

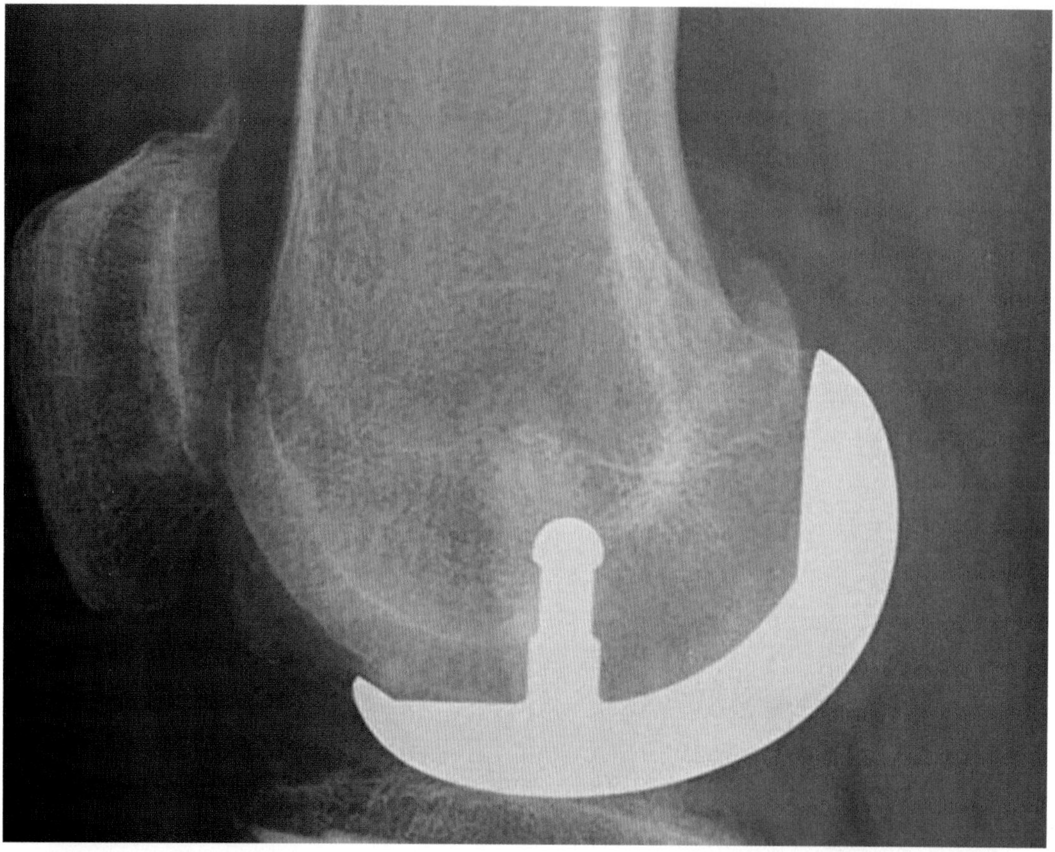

Fig. 6.23 A lateral radiograph of a femoral component with a single fixation lug that is parallel to the prosthetic posterior condyle. Anterior angulation of the drill used to prepare the lug hole promoted compression of the posterior bone–cement interface during cementing.

and outline the back edge of the metallic condyle to define and eventually remove any retained osteophytes or uncapped posterior condylar bone that could cause impingement on the tibial polyethylene during maximum flexion.

Final Preparation of the Tibial Component

Final sizing of the tibial component can now take place. In most systems, the tibia can be sized independently from the femur. One should use the largest size that does not overhang posteriorly or medially, in order to maximally cap the cut surface of the tibia and decrease focal forces that could promote loosening.

Earlier designs were symmetric so they could be used on either the medial or lateral compartment in both right and left knees. Asymmetric components are now the rule to allow maximal capping of the cut surface of the tibia. An asymmetric component also provides more polyethylene anteriorly and peripherally to accommodate the common anteromedial wear pattern in varus osteoarthritic knees. A custom designed tibial component will obviously maximize the tibial coverage (see Chapter 11).

Final mediolateral and rotational positioning of the tibial component is determined by a trial reduction. Congruency should be assessed with the knee in full extension. As noted previously, mediolateral congruency is altered by mediolateral placement of the femoral component. Rotational alignment is altered on the tibial side by changing the orientation of the resection along the tibial spine.

If the flexion space is too tight, the tibial component will lift off anteriorly or the femoral component will lift off from the distal femoral condylar resection. This can usually be resolved by applying a little more posterior tibial slope to the tibial resection as long as a total posterior slope of approximately 10 degrees is not exceeded. Alternatively, tightness in flexion can be resolved by downsizing the femoral component, which will require slightly more posterior condylar resection, thereby loosening the flexion gap. When doing so, the surgeon must be sure that the smaller component still provides adequate metal-to-plastic contact in full extension. If not, the same size femoral component is shifted anteriorly on the distal femur by resecting more posterior condyle and reorienting the fixation lugs to a more anterior location.

Cementing Components

Before the real components are cemented, they should be tested in the knee as if they were trials. It is important to do this because the lugs or fins of the real component may make insertion more difficult than that experienced with the lug-free trials. It is better to appreciate and resolve this difficulty before committing to the cementing process.

The tibial component is cemented first. Any lug holes or slots are packed under pressure with cement, and little or no cement is placed on the plateau itself (Fig. 6.24). The remaining cement is placed on the undersurface of the real tibial component (Fig. 6.25), which is inserted so that it makes contact posteriorly first. This prevents

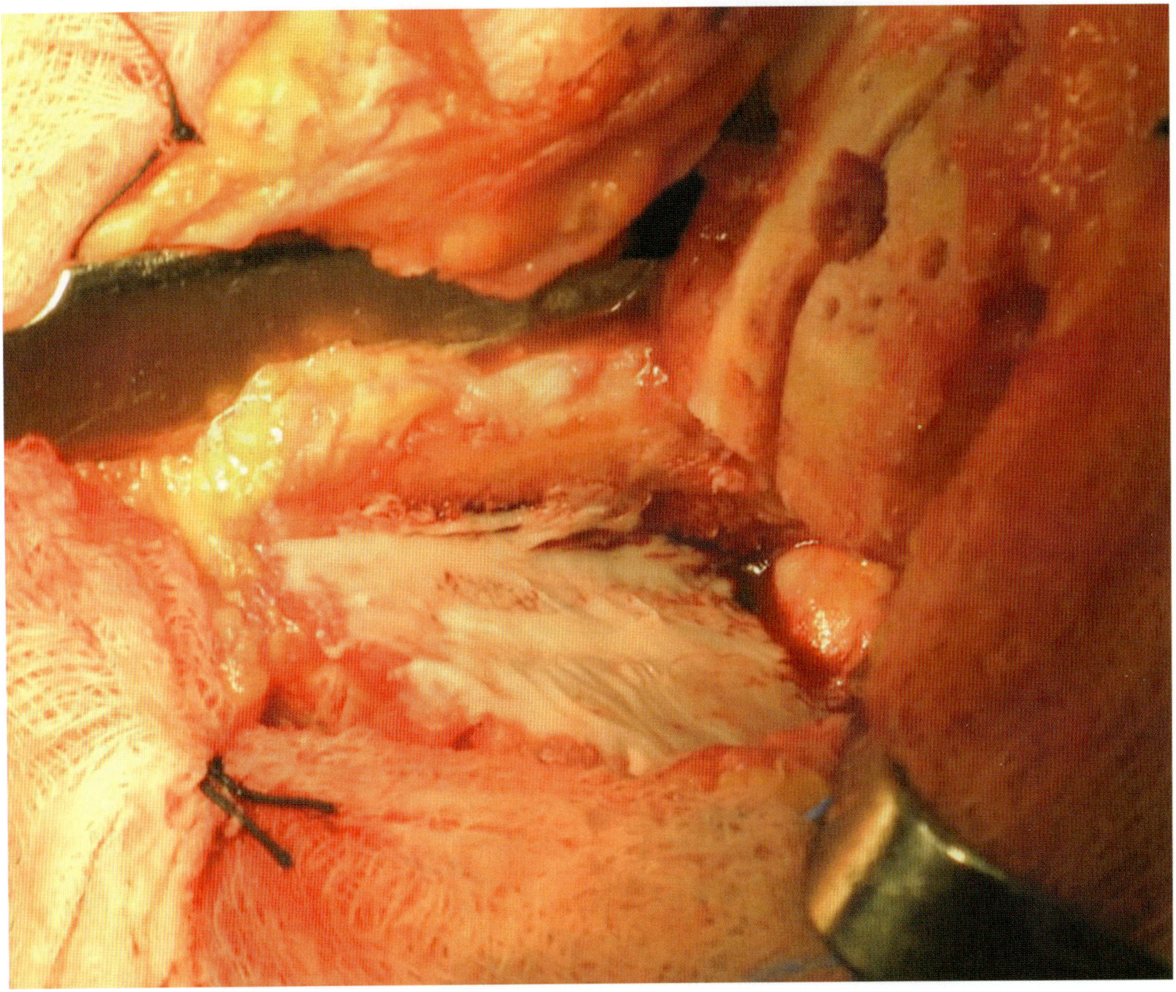

Fig. 6.24 An intraoperative photograph showing the tibial lug holes packed with cement and a thin film of cement smeared on the prepared tibial plateau.

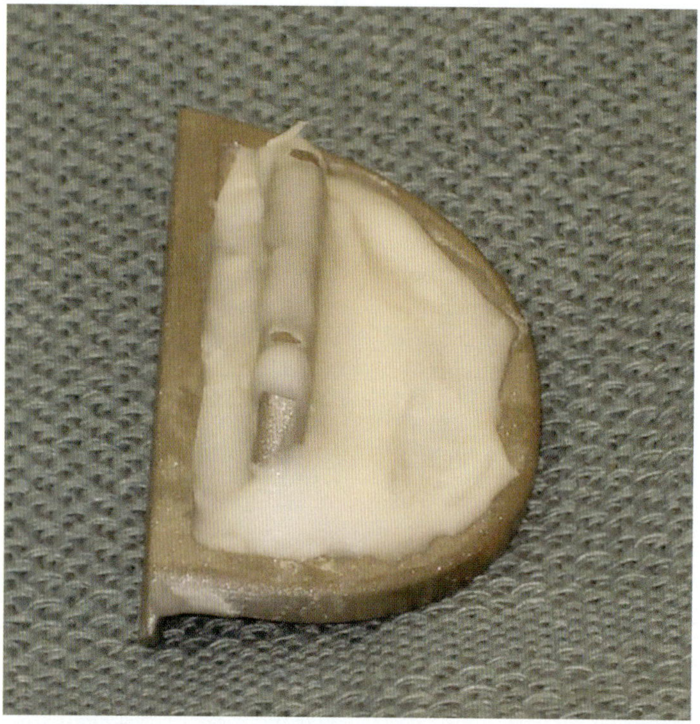

Fig. 6.25 An intraoperative photograph showing cement applied to the undersurface of the tibial component in preparation for cementation.

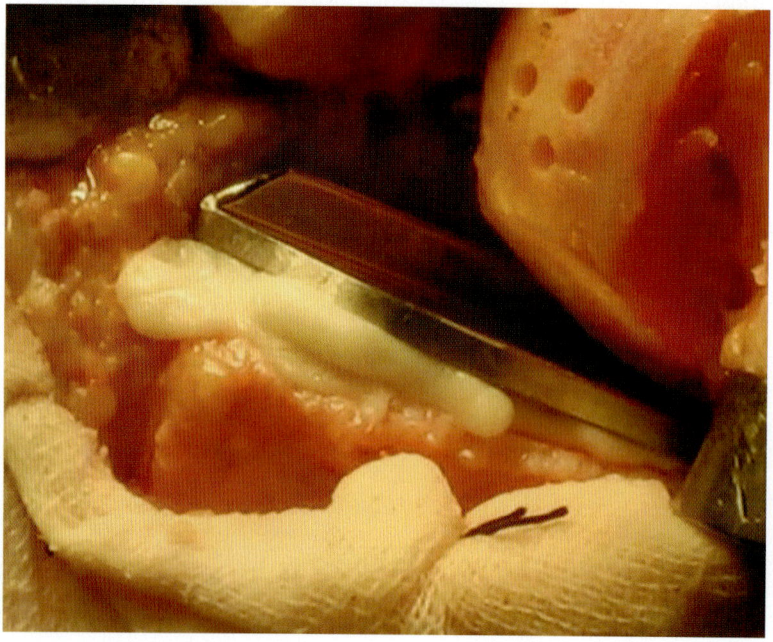

Fig. 6.26 If the tibial component is inserted with initial contact posteriorly, cement will be extruded anteriorly as it is fully seated.

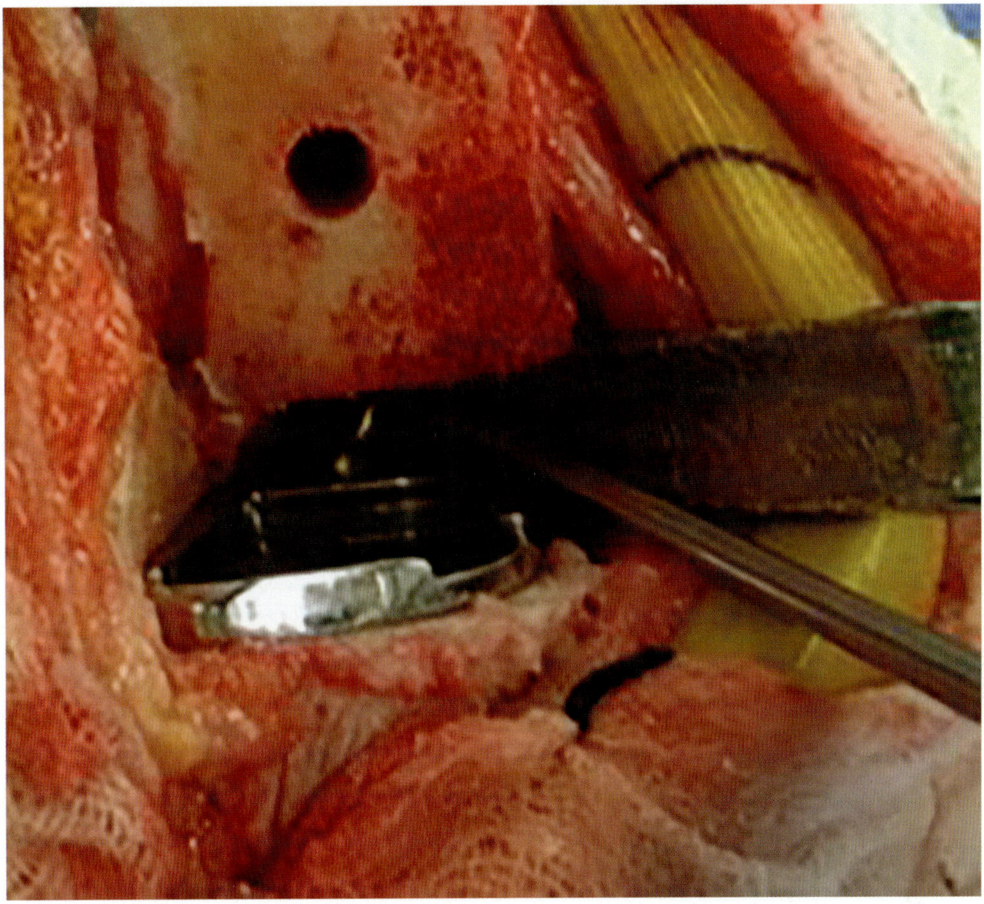

Fig. 6.27 A small angled curette is useful to access any extruded cement behind either the tibial or femoral component.

pushing any cement to the back of the knee and allows any extruded cement to come forward as the anterior aspect of the tibial component seats itself (Fig. 6.26). A small right-angled curette can be helpful in accessing and removing posterior cement from behind the femoral or tibial component (Fig. 6.27).

The femoral component is then cemented with a similar technique. Cement is placed on the distal femoral condyle and pressurized into any lug holes or slots. A thin film of cement is smeared onto the posterior condylar bone for cement intrusion there, and the remainder of the cement is placed on the inside of the femoral component (Fig. 6.28). If the tibial component is modular, a trial tibial insert is placed and the knee is slowly extended to pressurize the bone–cement interface. Any extruded cement is brought forward and removed. After terminal extension is achieved, the knee is rested in this position until full polymerization takes place. Flexing and extending the knee during the polymerization process may disrupt the prosthesis–cement or bone–cement interface and should be avoided.

After full polymerization, the knee is flexed and a tourniquet, if utilized, is deflated. If utilized during cementing, the trial tibial insert is removed and any further extruded cement is accessed. It is helpful to pass an instrument such as a straight pituitary rongeur along the tibial spine to be certain that no potential impingement exists between any retained bone or osteophyte. The knee should also be inspected peripherally for any extruded cement that could possibly break off at a later time. The real tibial insert is placed and the wound closed in the usual fashion.

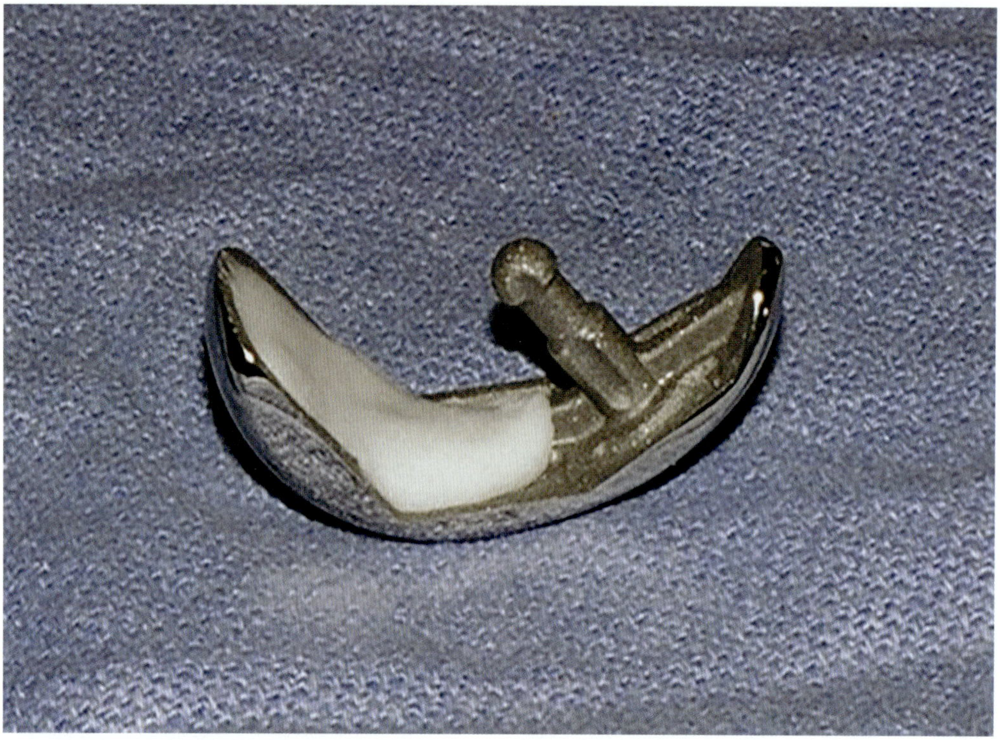

Fig. 6.28 If the femoral component has a recess in the posterior condyle, cement is placed there prior to insertion.

REFERENCES

1. Outerbridge RE. The aetiology of chondromalacia patellae. *J Bone Joint Surg Br*. 1961;43:752–757.
2. Berend KR, Berend ME, Dalury DF, Argenson JN, Dodd CA, Scott RD. Consensus statement on indications and contraindications for medial unicompartmental knee arthroplasty. *J Surg Orthop Adv*. 2015;24(4):252–256.
3. Repicci JA, Hartman JF. Minimally invasive unicondylar knee arthroplasty for the treatment of unicompartmental osteoarthritis: an outpatient arthritic bypass procedure. *Orthop Clin North Am*. 2004;35:201–216.
4. Brumby SA, Carrington R, Zayontz S, et al. Tibial plateau stress fracture: a complication of unicompartmental knee arthroplasty using 4 guide pins. *J Arthroplasty*. 2003;18: 809–812.
5. White SH, Ludkowski PF, Goodfellow JW. Anteromedial osteoarthritis of the knee. *J Bone Joint Surg Br*. 1991;73: 582–586.
6. McCallum JD, Scott RD. Duplication of medial erosion in unicompartmental knee arthroplasties. *J Bone Joint Surg Br*. 1995;77:726–728.

7

Mobile-Bearing Unicompartmental Knee Arthroplasty: Rationale and Surgical Technique

THE RATIONALE FOR A MOBILE-BEARING ARTICULATION

Mobile-bearing unicompartmental components were introduced in an attempt to increase the longevity of the prosthesis by maximizing the articular contact area, thereby reducing stress on the polyethylene and minimizing wear.[1] They might also reduce the rate of aseptic loosening in a conforming articulation. Stress across an articulation is related to the difference between the radius of curvature of the two articulating components. A round-on-flat articulation will promote high stresses. If the radii of curvature are identical, stress is minimized. It is also ideal if high contact can be maintained throughout the functional range of motion and be capable of accommodating to the normal anterior–posterior and rotational kinematics innate to each patient's individual knee. Although a flat-on-flat articulation with an identical (infinite) radius of curvature would fulfill the aforementioned criteria and provide minimal stress when precisely articulated, it could not maintain congruent contact throughout the range of motion and edge-loading would be inevitable. A round-on-round articulation with identical radii is ideal.

Fixed-bearing articulations with high conformity have been introduced in the past in an attempt to lower polyethylene stresses. As noted previously, the typical wear pattern of a varus osteoarthritic knee is anterior and peripheral[2] and the replaced knee wants to return to this wear pattern[3] (Fig. 7.1). When conforming fixed bearings were introduced to try to control this wear pattern, they suffered a higher-than-normal incidence of loosening because of the kinematic conflict that occurred (Fig. 7.2). It has been concluded, therefore, that fixed-bearing unicompartmental knee arthroplasty (UKA) articulations must be nonconforming, that is, round-on-relatively-flat. Maximally conforming UKAs must be mobile-bearing. They can provide maximum conformity on the topside of the articulation via the identical radius of curvature between the femoral component and the topside of the mobile-bearing insert while allowing adjustment to the anteromedial wear pattern via a flat-on-flat second articulation between the undersurface of the insert and the polished topside of the modular metallic tibial tray (Fig. 7.3). Other benefits of mobile-bearing metal-backed tibial components include that their modularity allows for a decreased inventory and for the potential for an isolated insert exchange if needed in the future. They also provide for a conservative composite component thickness of as little as 6 mm and for potential cementless fixation via the metallic undersurface. Early results employing cementless fixation in a mobile-bearing design have been favorable.[4]

SURGICAL TECHNIQUE

The basic principles of the surgical technique are similar to those described in Chapter 6 for fixed-bearing articulations: establish the flexion gap and then prepare the femur to equalize that gap.

The specific technique described later is taken in part from the online Oxford Partial Knee System surgical technique brochures[5] and adds some modifications from the authors' personal experiences. The authors defer to the Oxford brochure for any discrepancies. Instrumentation and specific technique will obviously evolve over time.

Preparation of the Tibia

The initial tibial resection should be as conservative as possible based on the preoperative templating described in Chapter 6 for fixed-bearing UKAs and documented in Fig. 6.2. After tibial resection is complete, the flexion gap is established using a spacer that reflects the composite

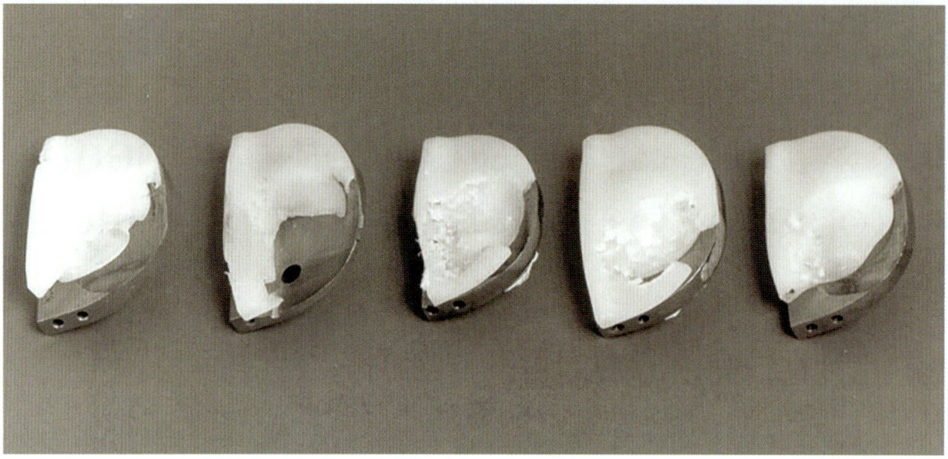

Fig. 7.1 Five retrieved failed tibial components all show replication of the patient's preoperative anteromedial wear pattern.

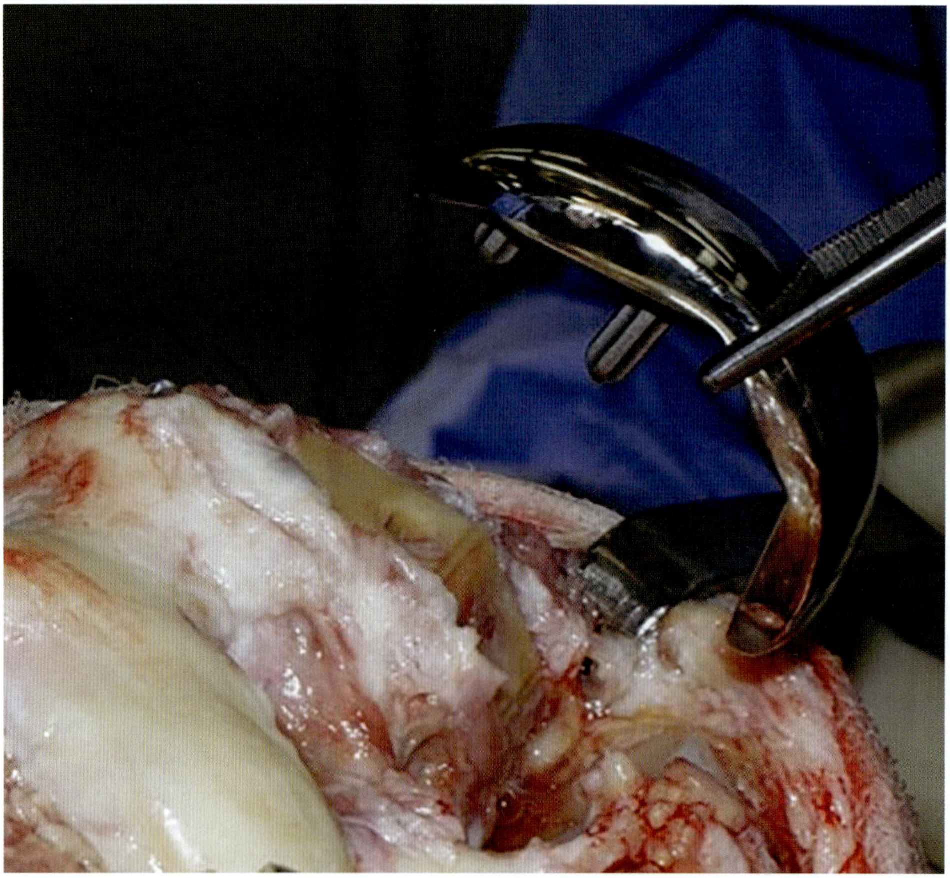

Fig. 7.2 Gross loosening of the femoral component is demonstrated in a fixed-bearing system that had a highly conforming tibiofemoral articulation.

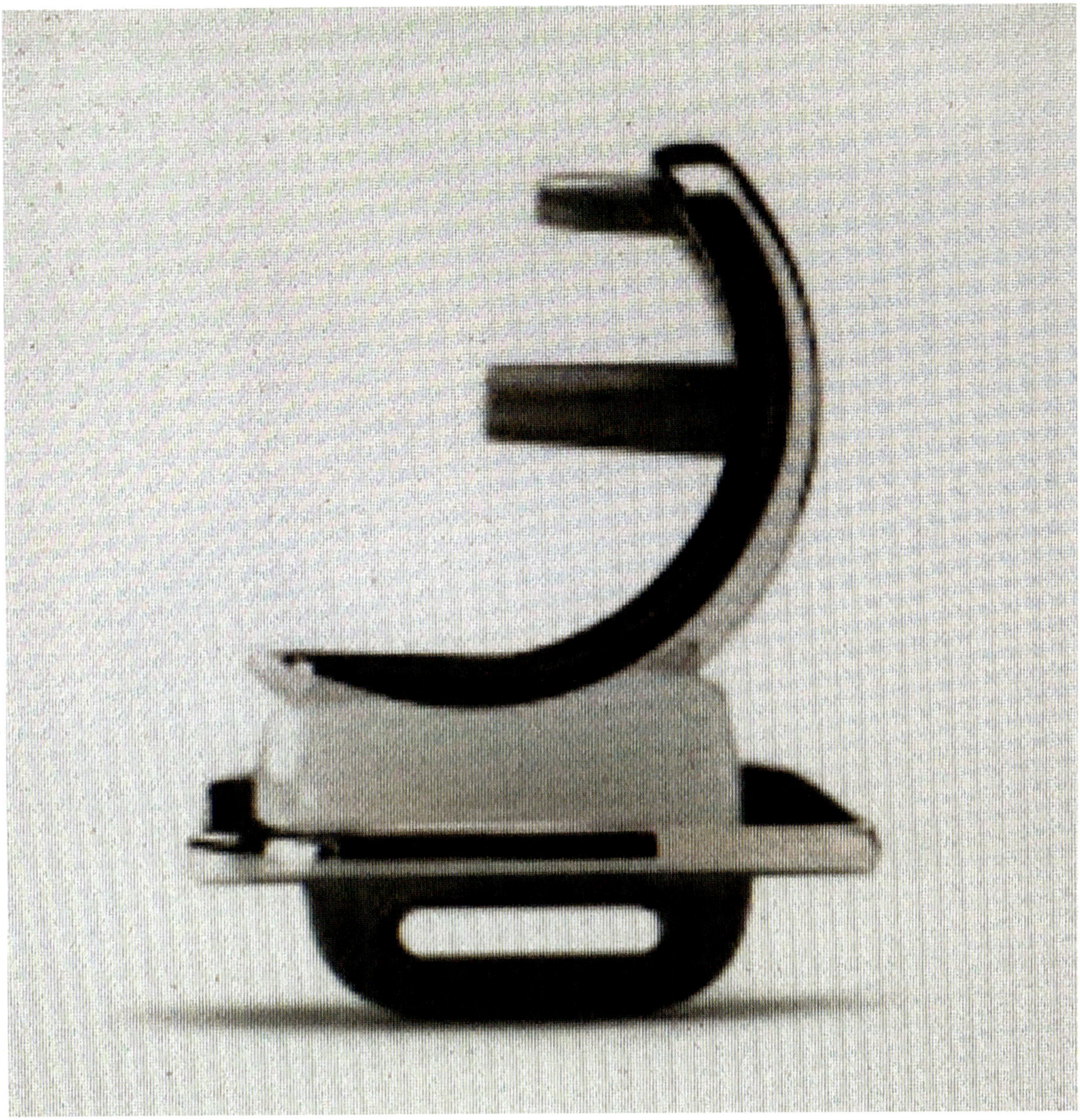

Fig. 7.3 The Oxford mobile-bearing partial knee replacement femoral and tibial components with a highly conforming round-on-round topside and flat-on-flat backside.

thickness of the appropriate tibial component. The thinnest and most conservative implantable composite thickness is 6 mm, but to avoid an overly tight flexion gap, a composite 7-mm trial thickness is recommended as a starting point (Fig. 7.4). If the flexion gap is smaller than 7 mm, it can be increased by skiving off any residual posterior condylar cartilage (as recommended in Chapter 6 for fixed bearings) unless the surgeon judges that the initial tibial resection was far too conservative, in which case the tibial resection is increased. Having established the flexion gap, attention is turned to the femoral preparation to equalize the extension gap.

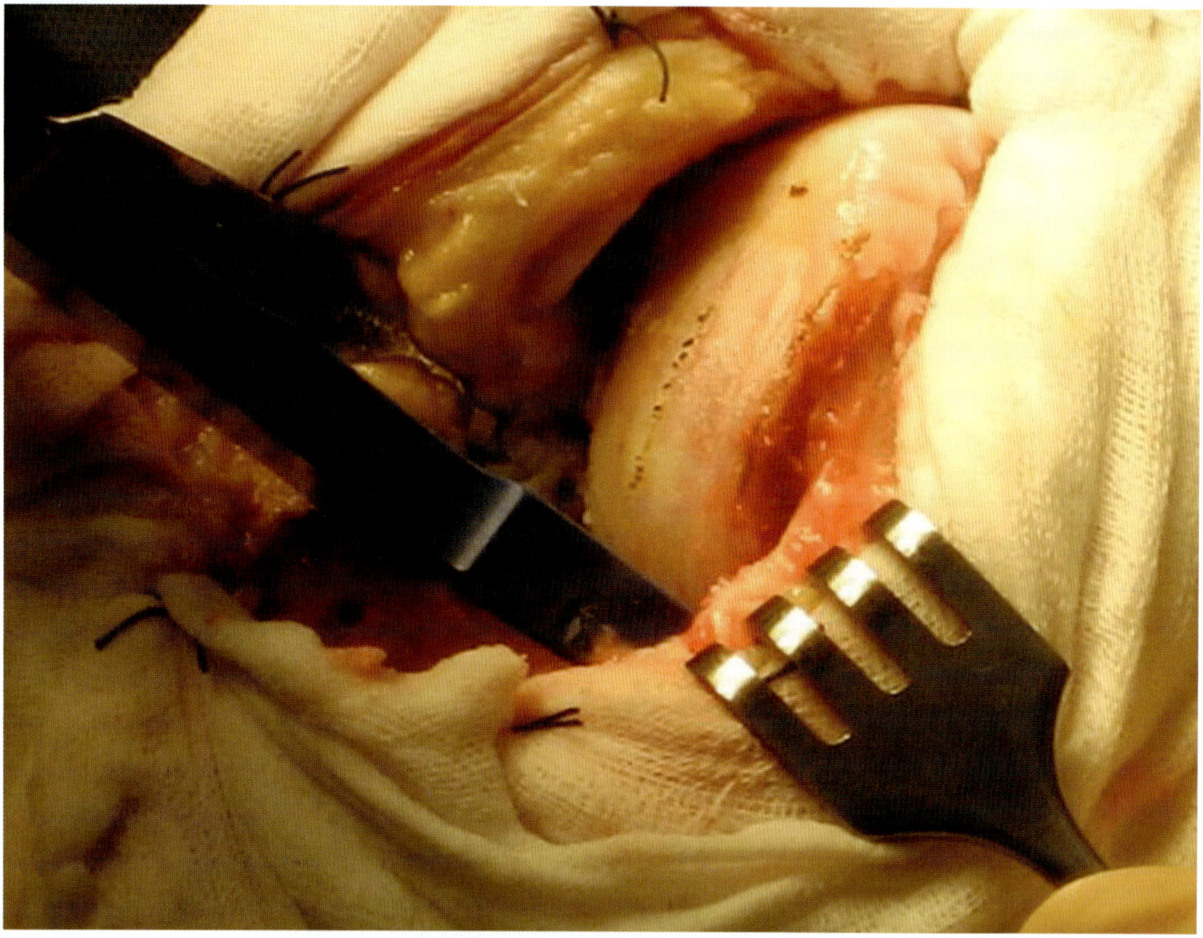

Fig. 7.4 The initial flexion gap is assessed using a 7-mm composite spacer.

Preparation of the Femur

As recommended for fixed-bearing UKA, the femoral anatomy is defined by removing intercondylar and peripheral osteophytes. In addition, it is helpful to define the true middle of the condyle by drawing a line down its center (Fig. 7.5). An intramedullary alignment rod is utilized to assist in preparation. A 4-mm hole is drilled approximately 5 mm above the origin of the posterior cruciate ligament and approximately 2 mm medial of center. The rod is gently and slowly introduced into the medullary canal to a depth of 8 to 10 cm. The femoral component size chosen by preoperative templating is confirmed by intraoperative measurement. The selected sizing jig is slid beneath the posterior condyle and its top surface aligned parallel to the alignment rod for correct flexion/extension orientation (Fig. 7.6). If it is sized correctly, its top rests approximately 5 mm posterior to the "tide-mark" (Fig. 7.7). Next the varus/valgus alignment of the jig (and femoral component) is established. The lateral border of the jig is adjusted so that it is parallel to the alignment rod (Fig. 7.8). It is important to avoid varus femoral component alignment and err toward slight valgus (Fig. 7.9). This decreases the chance of varus femoral orientation that could promote medial subluxation of the bearing (Fig. 7.10). With the sizing jig centered over the line drawn down the middle of the condyle, the lower of the two holes is drilled to prepare for the reaming spigots (this will also become the hole for the posterior of the two

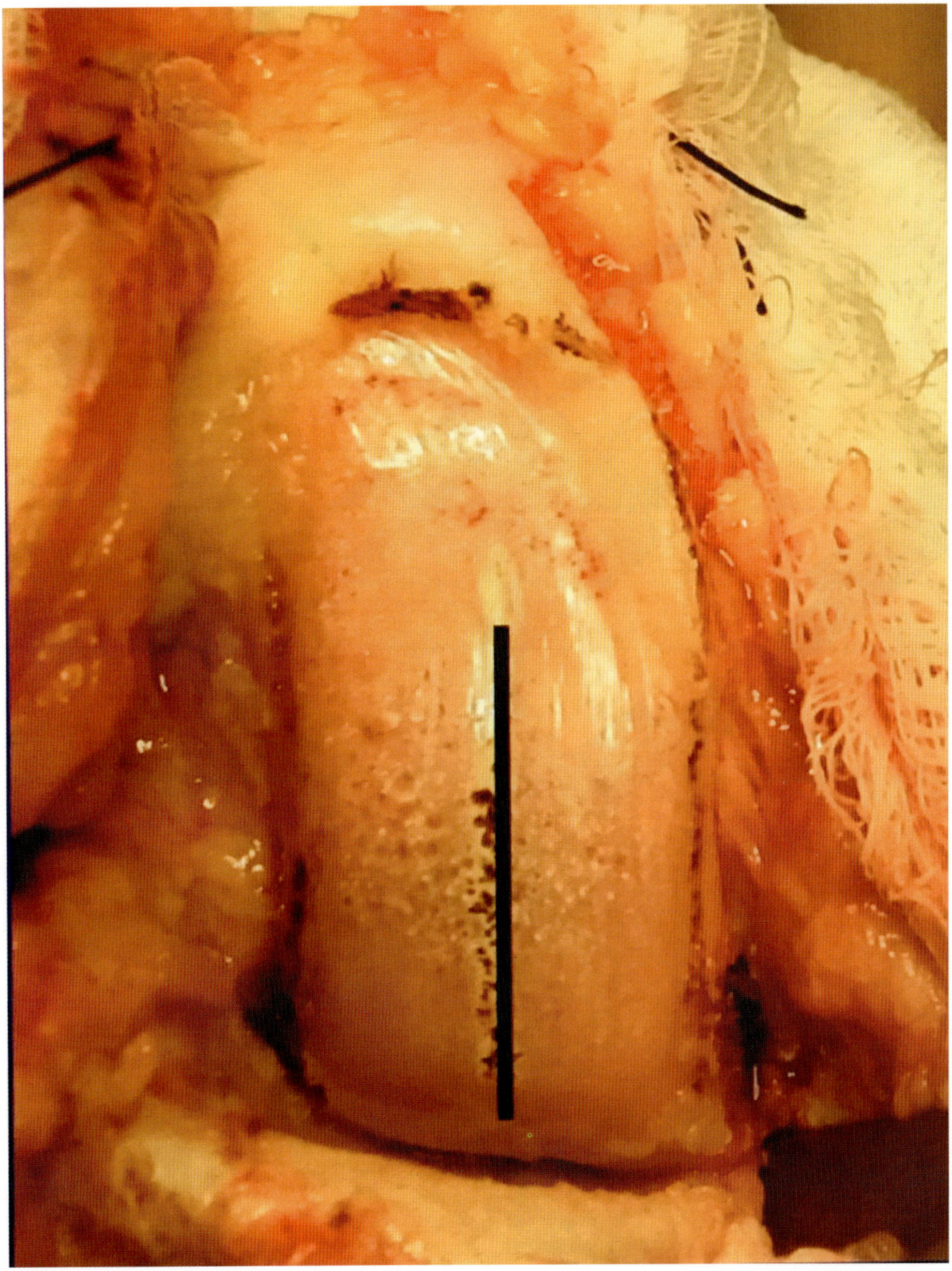

Fig. 7.5 The medial and lateral femoral osteophytes have been removed and the center of the condyle is defined with a marking pen or electrocautery.

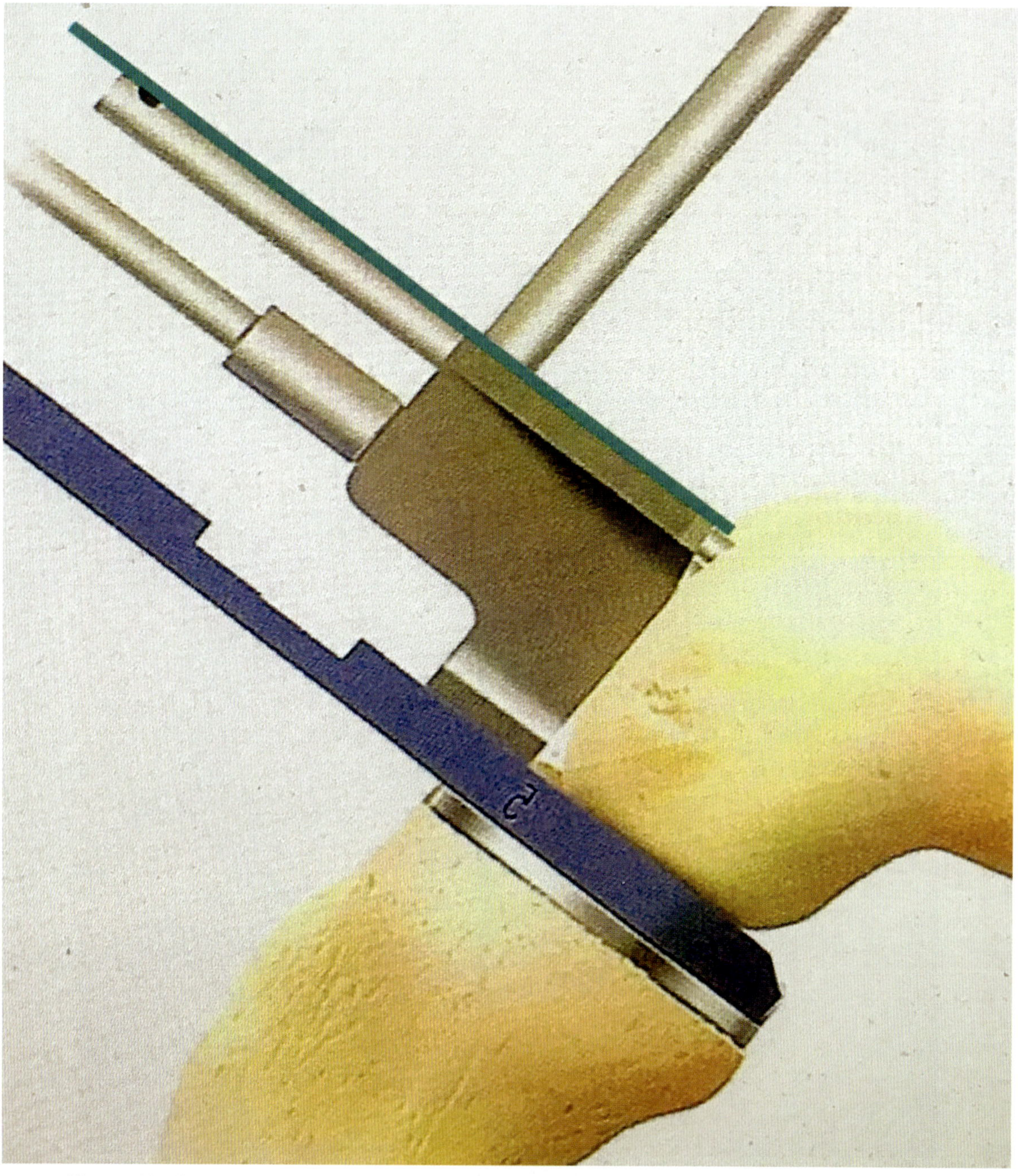

Fig. 7.6 The flexion/extension orientation of the femoral sizing jig should be parallel to the intramedullary alignment rod. *Oxford Partial Knee Replacement Surgical Technique, Zimmer Biomet.* Available at: https://www.zimmerbiomet.com/content/dam/zimmer-biomet/medical-professionals/000-surgical-techniques/knee/oxford-partial-knee-microplasty-instrumentation-surgical-technique.pdf.

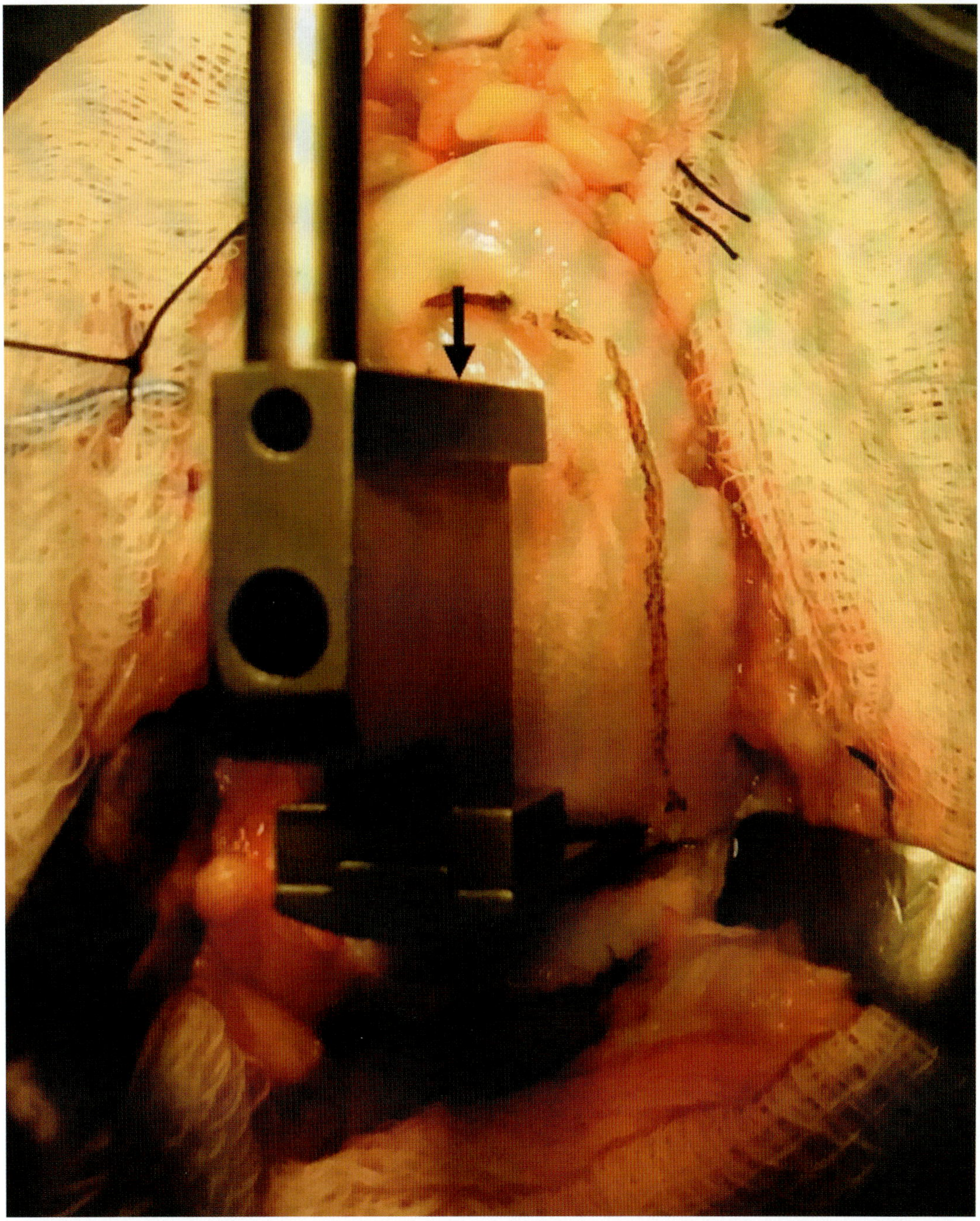

Fig. 7.7 The top of an appropriately sized femoral jig *(arrow)* usually lines up about 5 mm distal to the tide-mark (the junction between trochlear cartilage and condylar eburnated bone).

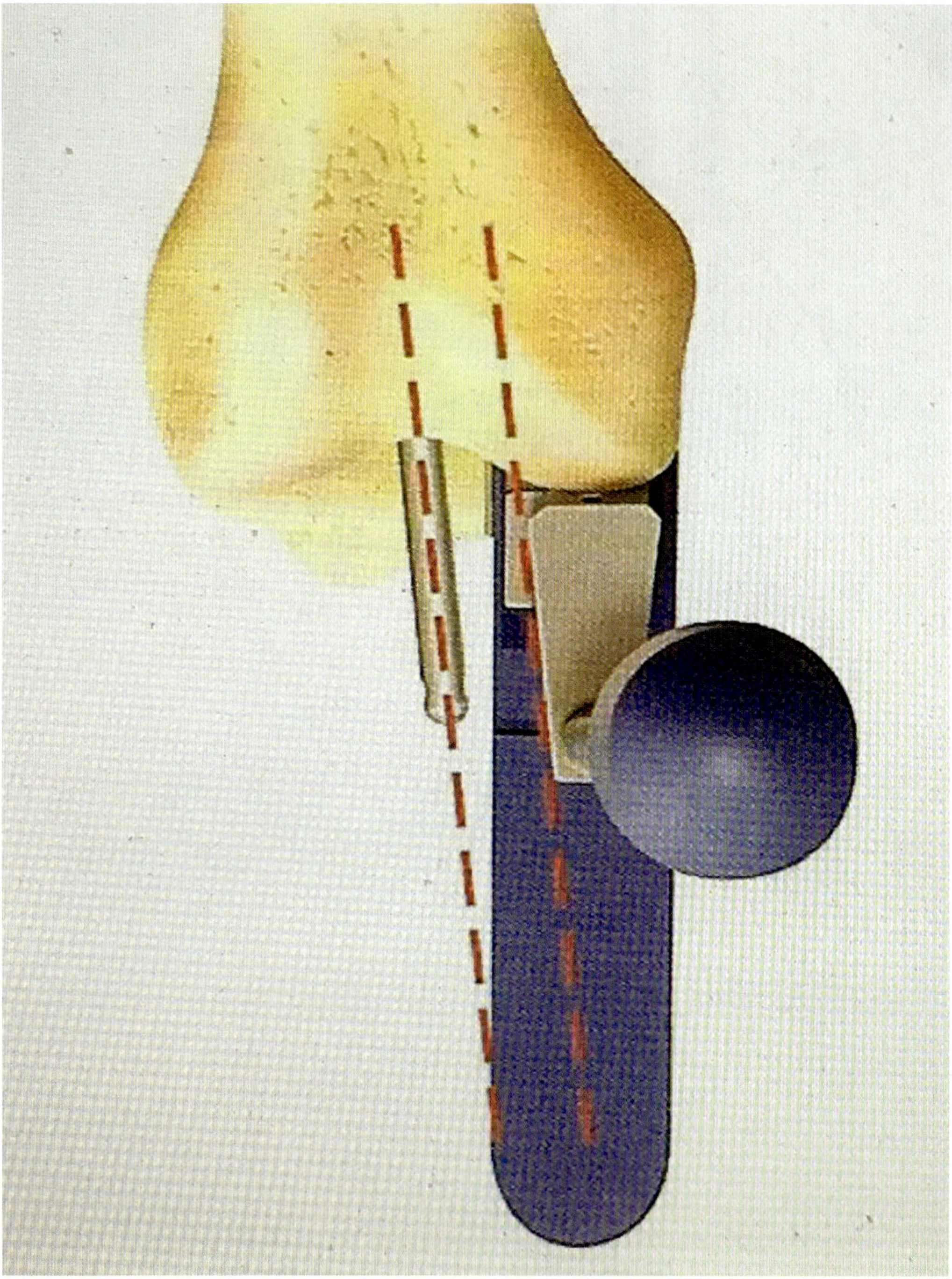

Fig. 7.8 Proper varus/valgus alignment of the femoral jig is achieved by lining up its medial border parallel with the intramedullary alignment rod. *Oxford Partial Knee Replacement Surgical Technique, Zimmer Biomet*. Available at: https://www.zimmerbiomet.com/content/dam/zimmer-biomet/medical-professionals/000-surgical-techniques/knee/oxford-partial-knee-microplasty-instrumentation-surgical-technique.pdf.

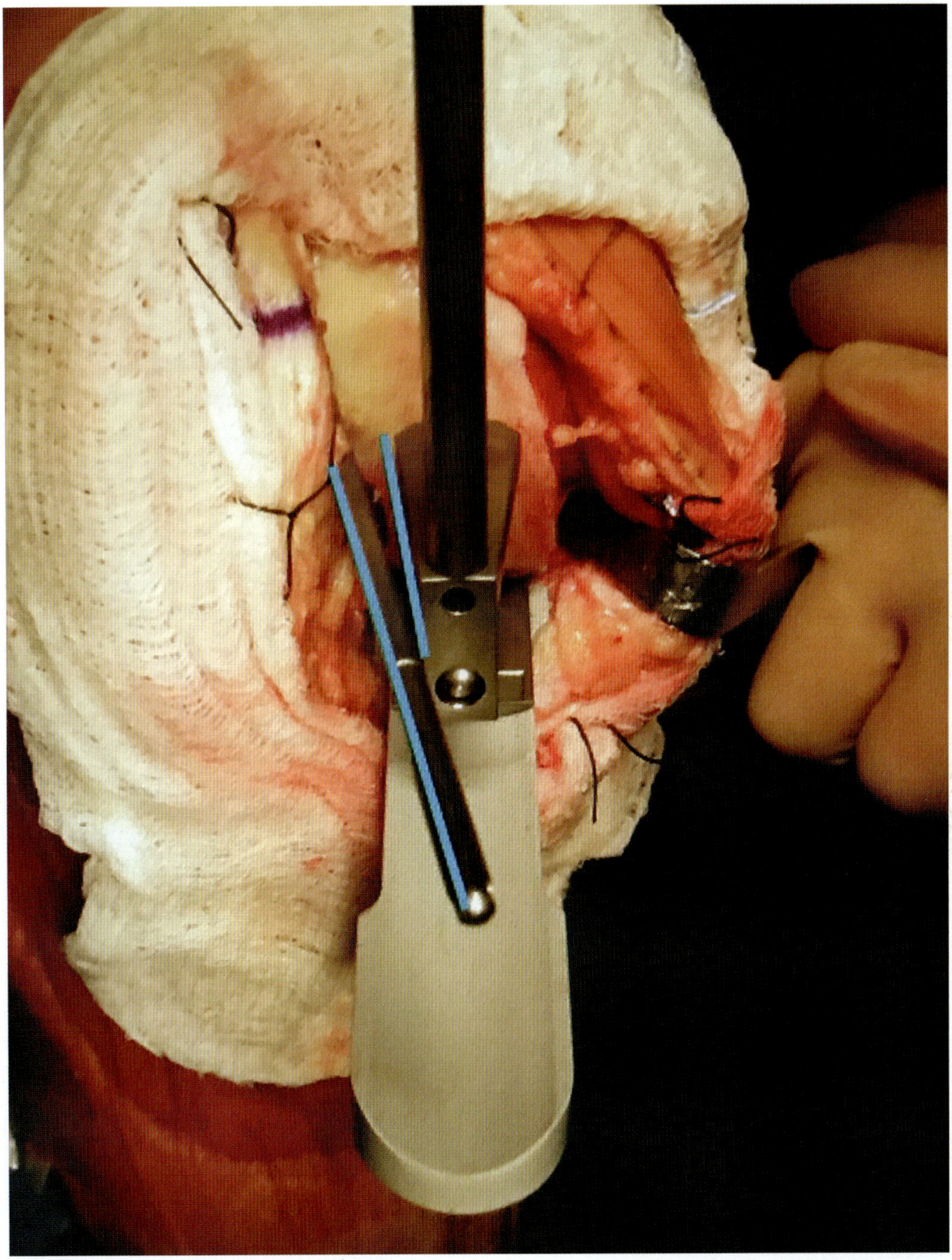

Fig. 7.9 As demonstrated in this photograph, the varus/valgus alignment chosen should err into valgus rather than varus (see Fig. 7.10).

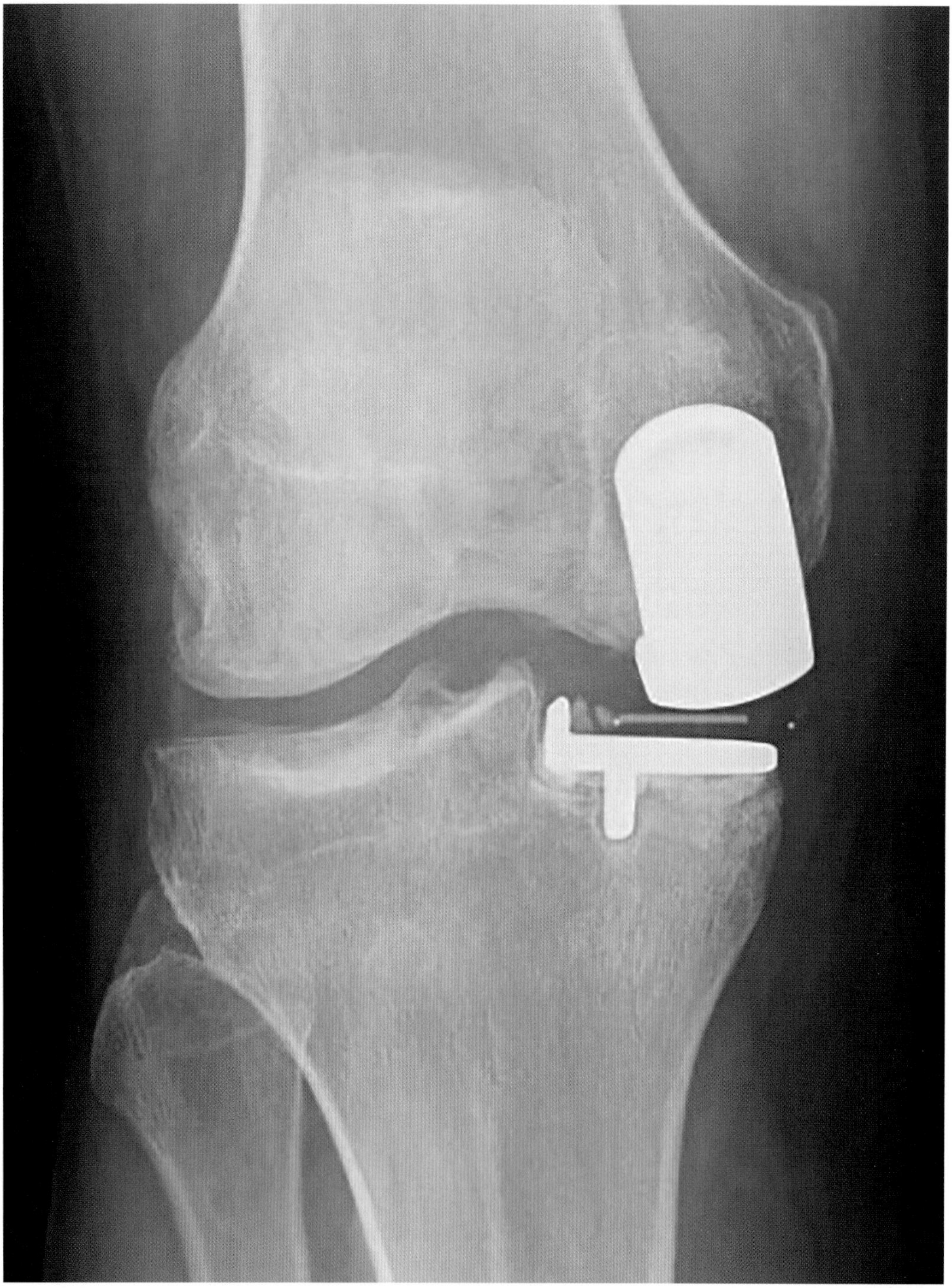

Fig. 7.10 A femoral component placed in varus can lead to medial subluxation of the mobile-bearing as demonstrated in this postoperative radiograph.

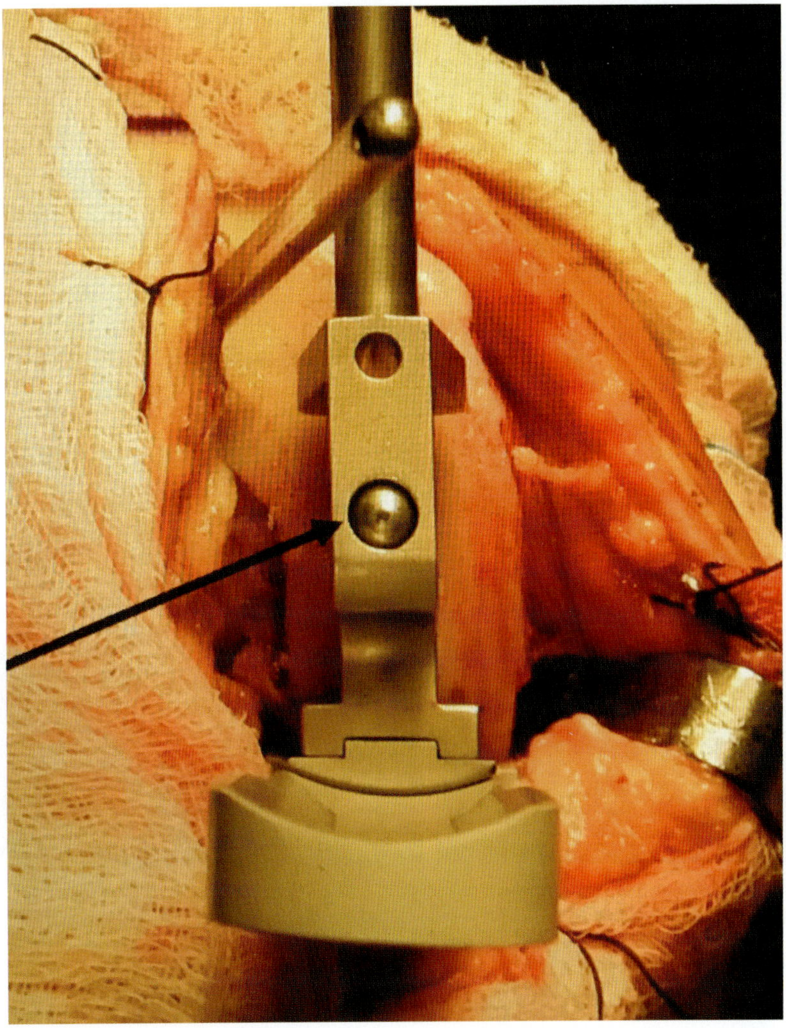

Fig. 7.11 To help secure the desired medial/lateral and rotational placement of the femoral jig, the lower hole is drilled first, centered over the line previously drawn on the condyle (see Fig. 7.5). A "zero" lug *(arrow)* is placed into this hole in order to secure this medial/lateral positioning and the jig is then rotated into proper rotational alignment to drill the second lug hole.

femoral component fixation lugs). A smooth spigot is tapped into this hole to secure the jig, which is then rotated until it is more or less perpendicular to the tibial resection (Fig. 7.11). The second more anterior hole is then drilled for the anterior fixation lug. Although this "neutral" femoral component rotation is ideal, if one errs it is better to err toward external femoral component rotation rather than internal rotation because an internally rotated femoral component will tend to force the bearing medially when the knee is in full extension (Fig. 7.12).

A newer generation of femoral preparation instruments is available to mechanically link the femoral jig to the intramedullary alignment rod and secure proper flexion/extension and varus/valgus alignment (Fig. 7.13). As noted earlier, instrumentation will continue to evolve but the surgical principles will likely remain unchanged.

The posterior condylar resection can now be performed parallel to the undersurface of the sizing jig. Some guides have cutting slots to direct the saw. If the guide is not slotted, the surgeon should err toward diverging this cut rather than converging it to assure maximum contact

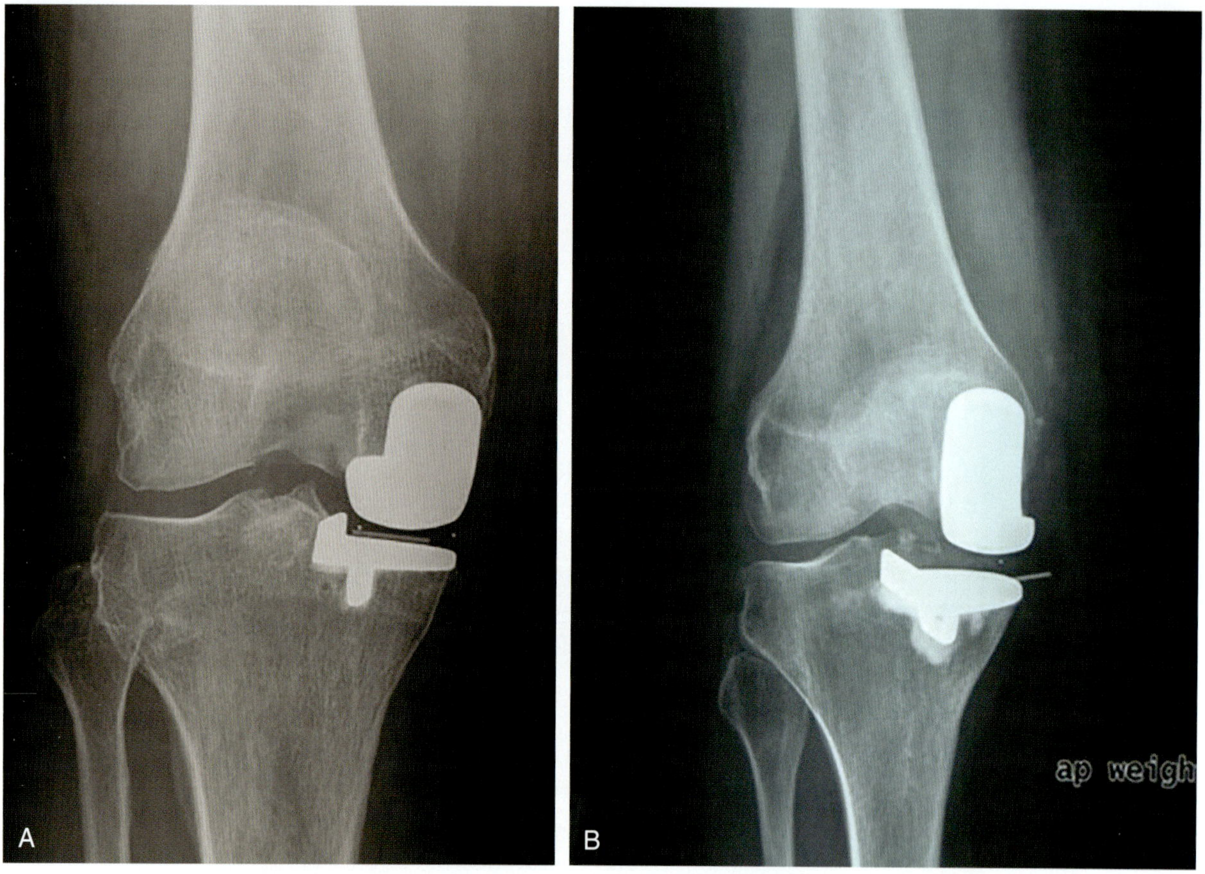

Fig. 7.12 (A) As shown in this postoperative radiograph, some external rotation of the femoral component is acceptable as it keeps the mobile tibial bearing well-located on the tibial tray. (B) As shown in this postoperative radiograph, internal rotation of the femoral component should be avoided because it can lead to medial subluxation of the bearing.

between the metallic posterior condyle and the posterior condylar bone.

The reaming of the femoral condyle can now commence to equalize the extension gap with the flexion gap. The initial ream is with a 0 (zero) spigot, after which a trial femoral component is mated with the trial tibial component. If the extension gap is too tight and does not allow full extension, progressively more sequential femoral reaming is performed until the gaps are equalized. Spigots are available that are labelled from 1 to 7. The number of each spigot reflects the increased depth of femoral reaming that will be achieved relative to the initial ream of "0." The reaming will normally create a recess in the anterior condylar femoral cartilage that prohibits the anterior aspect of the mobile-bearing from impinging in full extension. If the recess is insufficient, a gouge can be used to enlarge this "divot" and further relieve any impingement (Fig. 7.14).

Implantation

Cementing of the real components progresses as described for fixed bearings in Chapter 6. A trial spacer is utilized to pressurize the interfaces, and the knee is held in 20 degrees of flexion until polymerization is complete. At this point, the spacer is removed and any extruded cement is excised. The real mobile-bearing insert is pushed

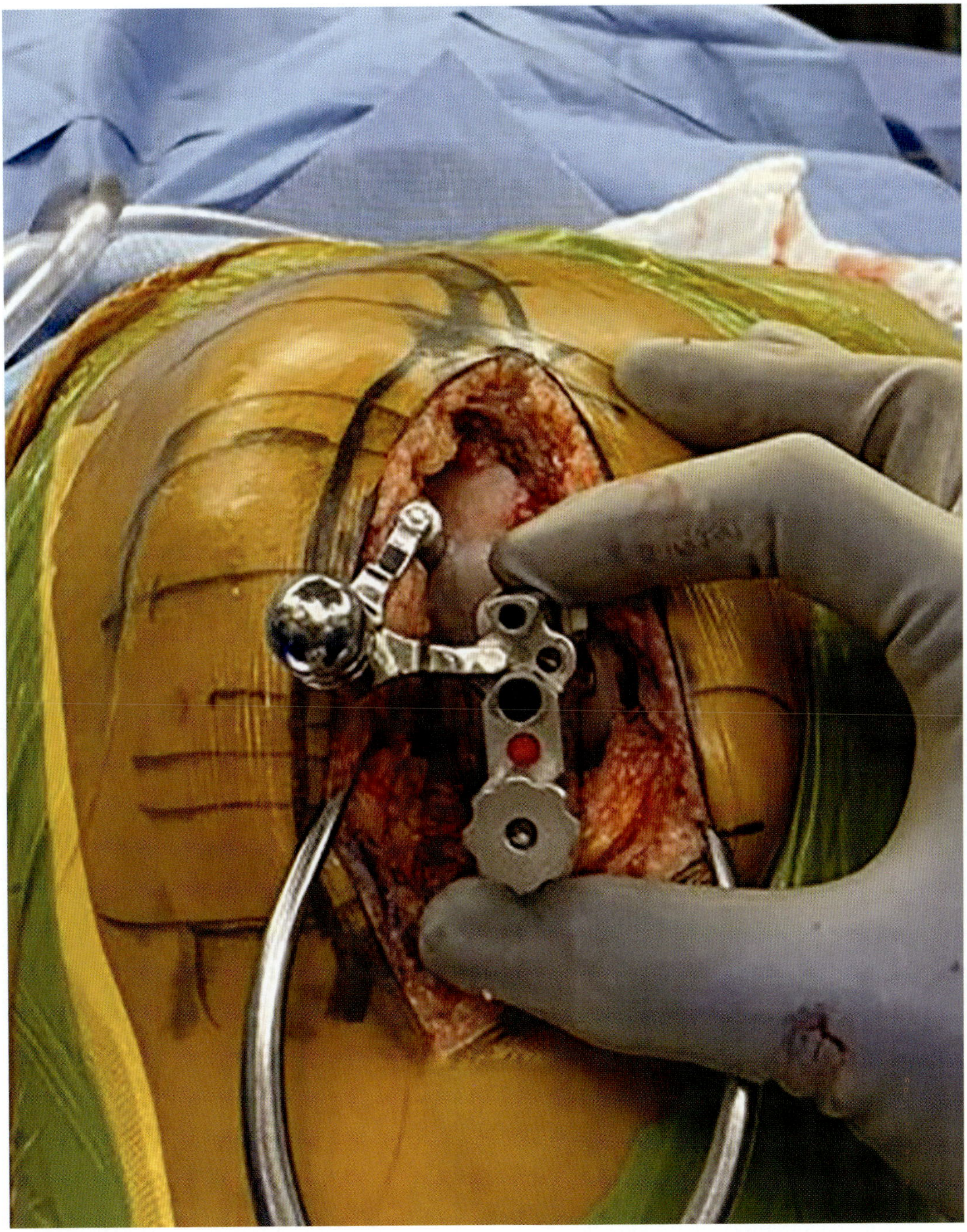

Fig. 7.13 Newer instrumentation mechanically links the femoral preparation jig to the intramedullary alignment rod to help establish proper flexion/extension and varus/valgus alignment.

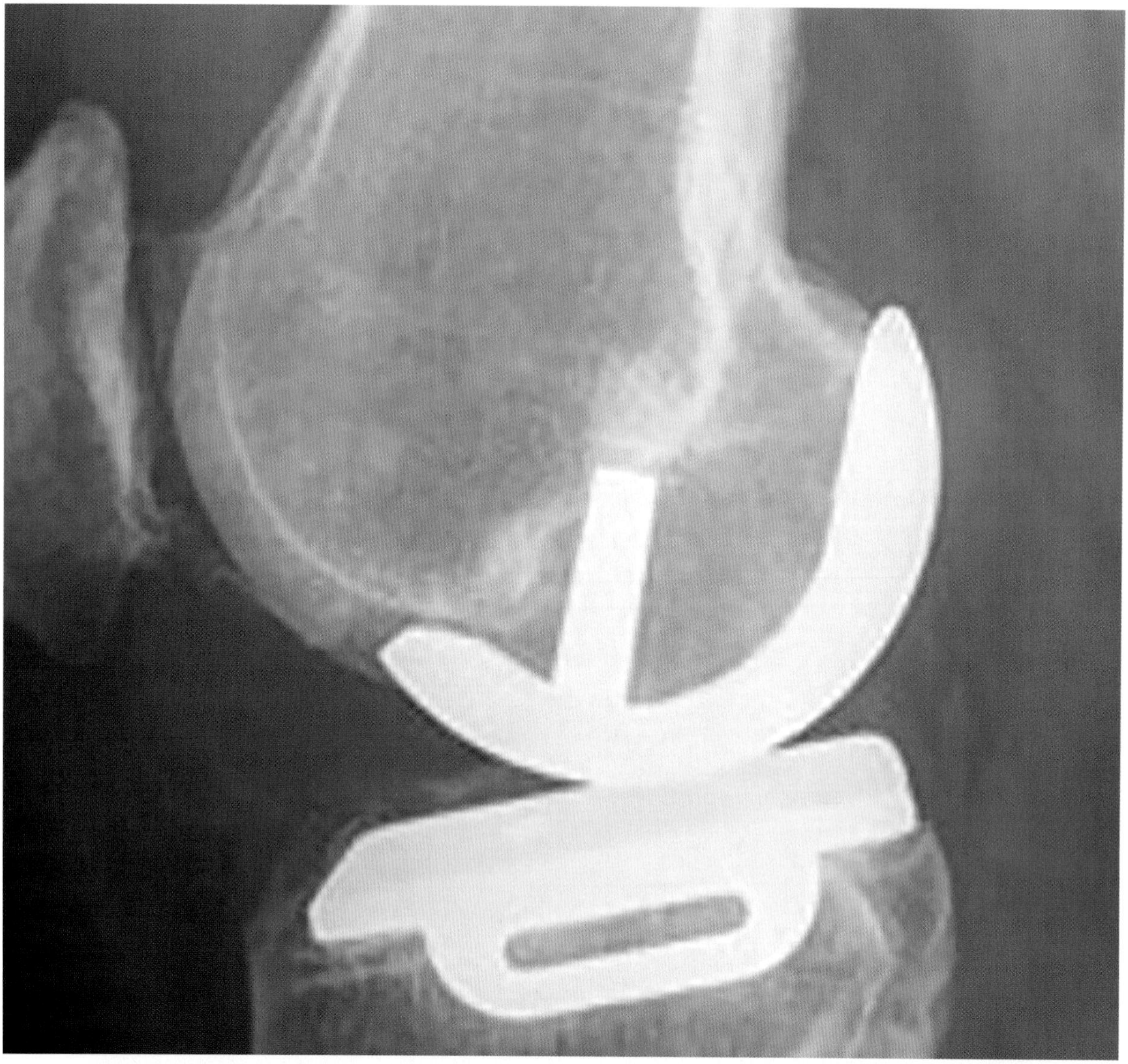

Fig. 7.14 The femoral reaming process usually results in a "divot" anterior to the leading edge of the femoral component. This relieves potential impingement of the tibial bearing on the femoral condyle in full extension. If necessary, the surgeon can enlarge this divot using a gouge.

into place using thumb pressure with the knee flexed approximately 80 degrees. If the flexion gap is appropriately tensioned, "significant" thumb pressure is required.

Under ideal circumstances, a well-executed arthroplasty will show a conservative tibial resection, correction of the preoperative varus deformity into mild anatomic valgus (slight mechanical varus), and congruent alignment between the femoral and tibial components (Fig. 7.15). Slight mechanical varus will minimize the chance of late secondary degeneration of the lateral compartment.

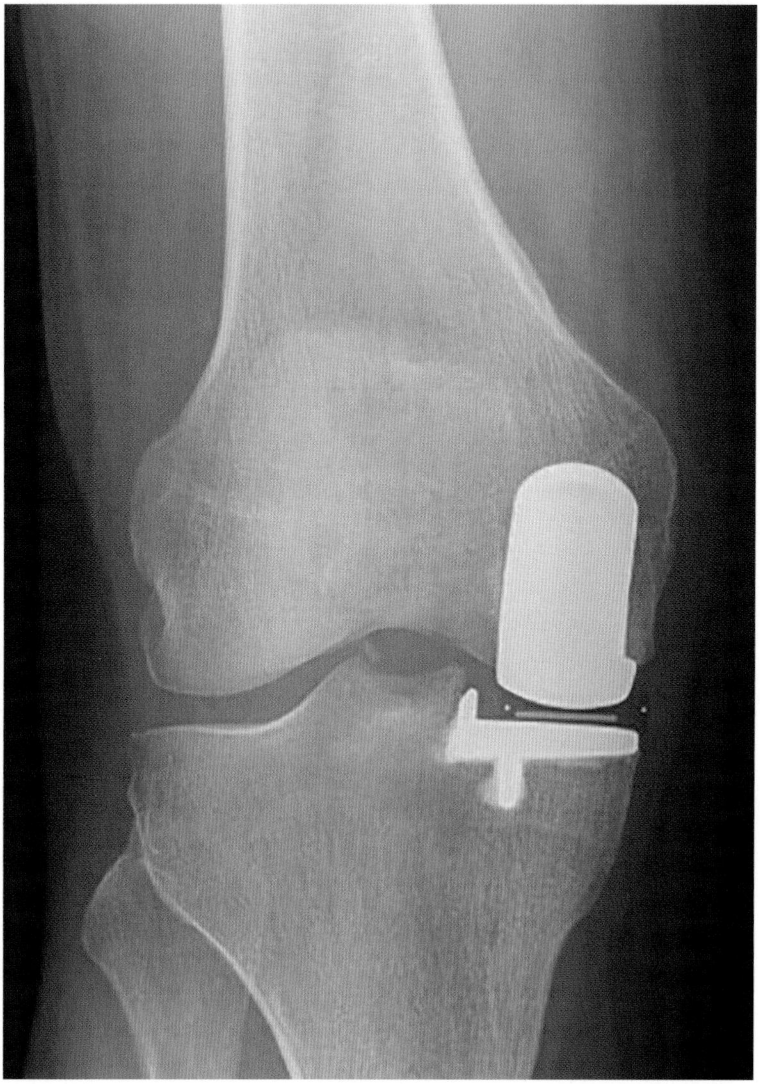

Fig. 7.15 A postoperative radiograph of a well-aligned mobile-bearing arthroplasty shows a conservative tibial resection, appropriate correction of the varus deformity, and good congruency between the articulating components.

REFERENCES

1. Murray DW, Goodfellow JW, O'Connor JJ. The Oxford medial unicompartmental arthroplasty: a ten-year survival study. *J Bone Joint Surg Br*. 1988;80-B(6):983–989.
2. White SH, Ludkowski PF, Goodfellow JW. Anteromedial osteoarthritis of the knee. *J Bone Joint Surg Br*. 1991;73:582–586.
3. McCallum JD, Scott RD. Duplication of medial erosion in unicompartmental knee arthroplasties. *J Bone Joint Surg Br*. 1995;77:726–728.
4. Campi S, Pandit H, Hooper G, et al. Ten-year survival and seven-year functional results of cementless Oxford unicompartmental knee replacement: a prospective consecutive series of our first 1000 cases. *Knee*. 2018;25(6):1231–1237.
5. *Oxford Partial Knee Replacement Surgical Technique, Zimmer Biomet*. Available at: https://www.zimmerbiomet.com/content/dam/zimmer-biomet/medical-professionals/000-surgical-techniques/knee/oxford-partial-knee-microplasty-instrumentation-surgical-technique.pdf.

8

Lateral Compartment Arthroplasty

INDICATIONS

The indications for lateral unicompartmental knee arthroplasty (UKA) are similar to those for medial UKA. The incidence of its need, however, is much less than that for medial replacement. In most experienced UKA practices, lateral arthroplasty comprises about 10% of UKAs.

The patient is more likely to be female and will present with a valgus knee alignment along with lateral knee pain and radiographic changes limited to the lateral compartment. The anterior cruciate ligament (ACL) should be intact. The radiographic presence of chondrocalcinosis is more frequent in lateral versus medial disease and does not contraindicate UKA as long as there is no history of chronic or recurrent active synovitis. As the wear pattern in lateral osteoarthritis is posterior on both the femur and the tibia, a standard standing anteroposterior (AP) radiograph may still show a joint space in end-stage disease. A posteroanterior (PA) standing flexed view may be necessary to demonstrate the loss of joint space and should be obtained routinely (Fig. 8.1).

For the knee to be a candidate for lateral UKA, deformity should be less than 12 degrees of anatomic valgus alignment (or less than 5 to 7 degrees of mechanical axis valgus). Deformity beyond this is often associated with medial collateral ligament laxity, which is a contraindication to lateral UKA (Fig. 8.2).

SURGICAL PRINCIPLES

The procedure for a lateral UKA is technically more difficult than for medial UKA, in part because it is performed less frequently. Patellar impingement is more likely because the patella normally favors articulating on the lateral rather than the medial femoral condyle in high flexion, making it critical that the leading edge of the femoral component is recessed into the trochlear cartilage at surgery.

As opposed to the wear pattern in medial osteoarthritis, which is anterior and peripheral,[1] the wear pattern in lateral disease is posterior. This fact makes it even more important that the ACL is intact and functioning and also leads to the recommendation that little or no posterior slope be applied to the tibial resection to discourage posterior tracking of the femoral component on the tibial component polyethylene (Fig. 8.3). This tendency for posterior wear and component tracking also means that mobile-bearing articulations are discouraged from being used in lateral arthroplasty to avoid posterior subluxation or dislocation of the bearing.[2] Clinically, a physical examination can elicit bony crepitus if the knee is gently ranged between 30 and 60 degrees of flexion while a valgus stress is being applied. This posterior wear pattern also explains why some patients with significant lateral arthritis have acceptable standing and walking tolerance but have major complaints when their knee is loaded in flexion, such as when negotiating hills or stairs.

SURGICAL TECHNIQUE

The surgical approach for lateral UKA can be medial or lateral. Advantages of a lateral incision include direct access and a shorter incision, as well as more rapid return of quadriceps function given decreased tendon violation.[3,4] Advantages of a medial arthrotomy include the opportunity to thoroughly evaluate the remainder of the joint for the appropriateness of the procedure and to intraoperatively convert to a total knee arthroplasty if necessary.[5] Although conversion is still possible through a lateral approach, it is technically much more demanding. Furthermore, if revision is required in the future, the medial skin incision and medial arthrotomy can be re-utilized for easy exposure. A prior lateral incision could possibly compromise wound healing if a new medial

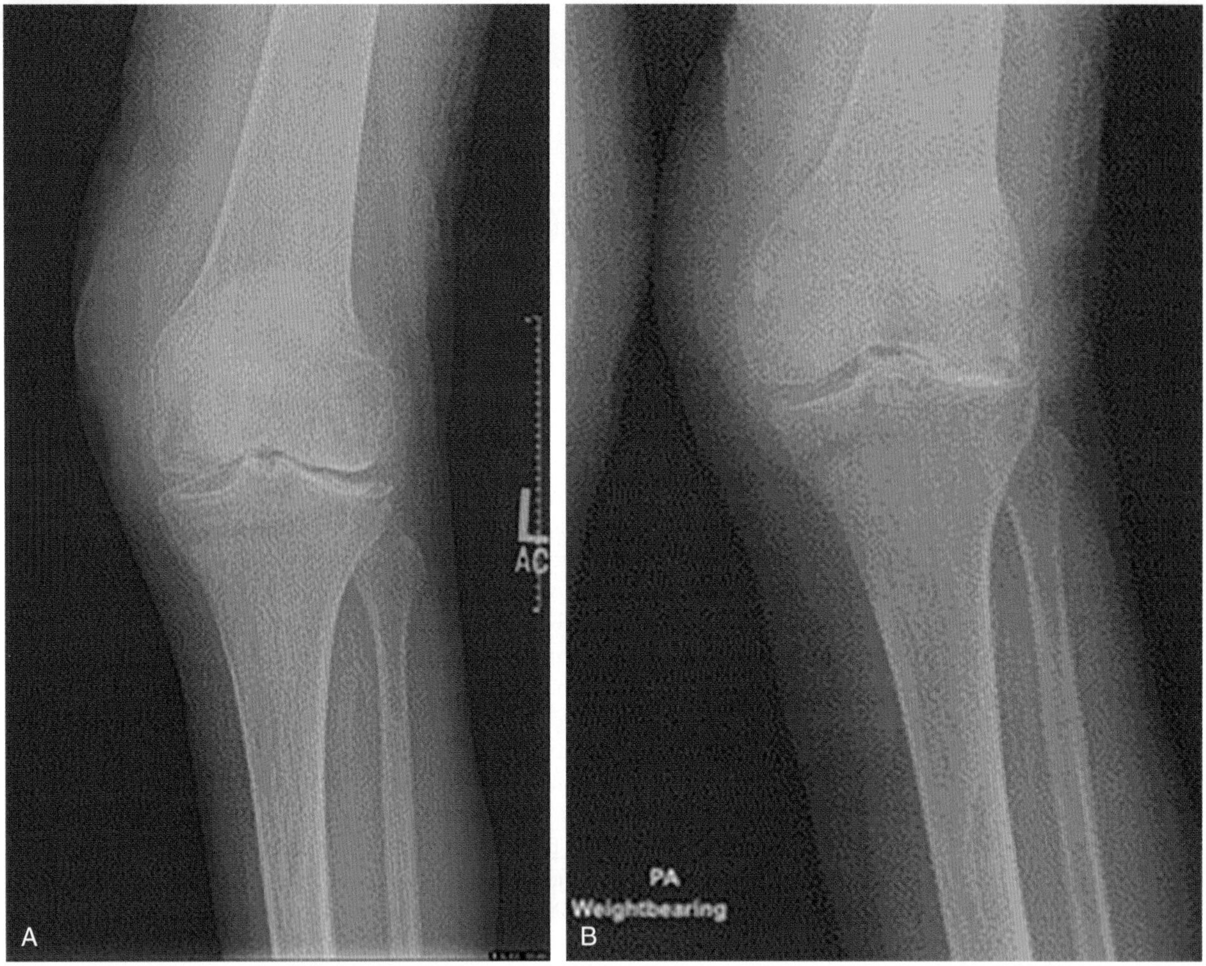

Fig. 8.1 (A) A standard standing AP radiograph may still show a lateral joint space in end-stage disease because the loss of cartilage is often posterior rather than distal. (B) A PA standing, partially flexed, knee radiograph in the same patient reveals the joint space loss. *AP,* Anteroposterior; *PA,* posteroanterior.

incision for the revision devascularizes the intervening skin bridge. For that reason, if a lateral arthrotomy is utilized, the skin incision should be midline if a medial approach is required in the future for a revision procedure.[4]

Medial Approach

For a medial arthrotomy, the skin incision can be short. As the arthrotomy approaches the anterior horn of the medial meniscus, the dissection is taken laterally, anterior to the coronary ligament, to avoid derangement of the medial meniscus.[5] The patella is subluxed or everted and the knee flexed. Enough of the fat pad is removed from the anterior aspect of the tibia to expose its anterior aspect for the tibial resection. An incision is made at the midcoronal plane of the lateral plateau just outside the lateral meniscus for placement of a bent Hohmann retractor. Moist wound towels can protect the subcutaneous tissue and the medial compartment throughout the remainder of the procedure (Fig. 8.4).

The distal femur often has residual cartilage (Fig. 8.5) that should be removed before the distal femoral bone resection to avoid underresection of the distal condyle that might hinder recessing the leading edge of a fixed-bearing femoral component (Fig. 8.6). This increased distal femoral resection calls for a very conservative initial tibial resection (Fig. 8.7) to avoid the need for very thick tibial

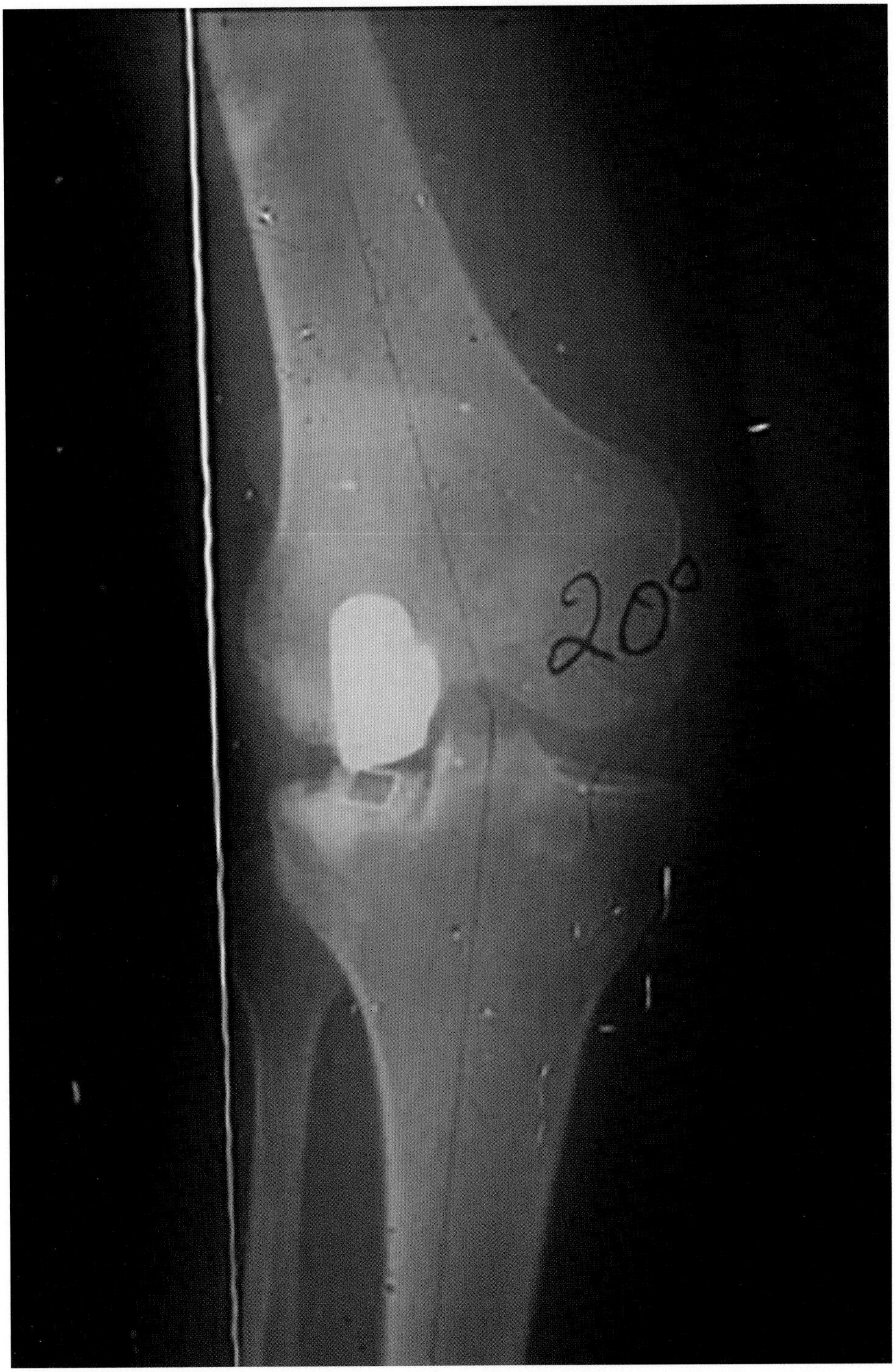

Fig. 8.2 A lateral unicompartmental knee arthroplasty cannot restore stability to a knee with preoperative medial collateral ligament laxity, as shown in this standing postoperative radiograph.

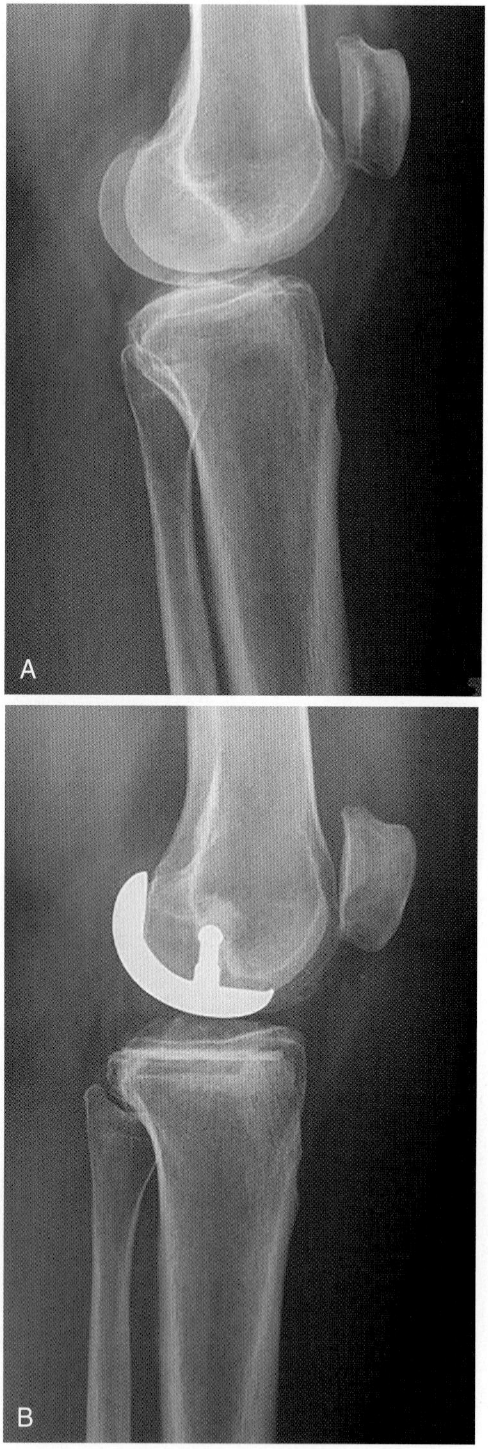

Fig. 8.3 (A) A preoperative lateral radiograph showing the extent of posterior slope in the lateral compartment that is typical in a patient with isolated lateral osteoarthritis. (B) A postoperative lateral radiograph showing minimal posterior slope applied to the tibial resection.

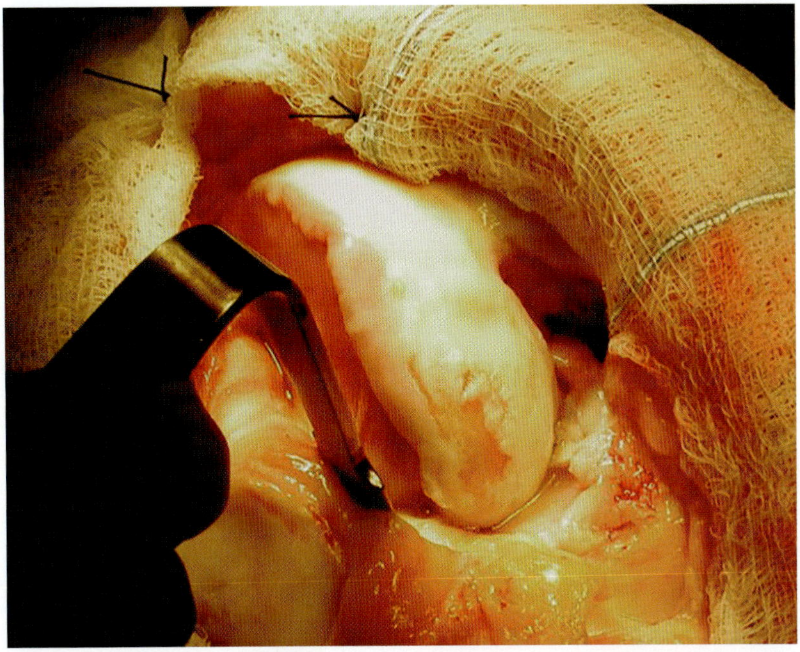

Fig. 8.4 Intraoperative exposure achieved by a medial arthrotomy for a lateral arthroplasty. The soft tissues and medial compartment are protected by moist wound towels.

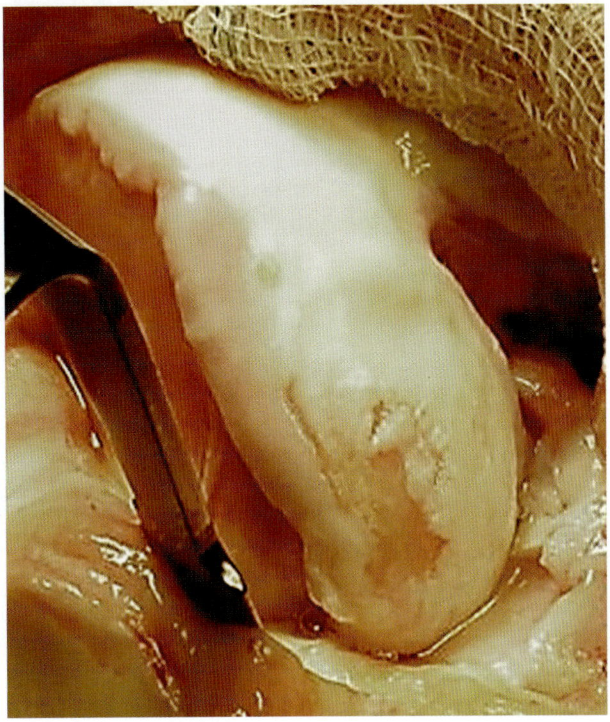

Fig. 8.5 An intraoperative photograph showing retained distal femoral cartilage and the posterior wear pattern typical of lateral osteoarthritis.

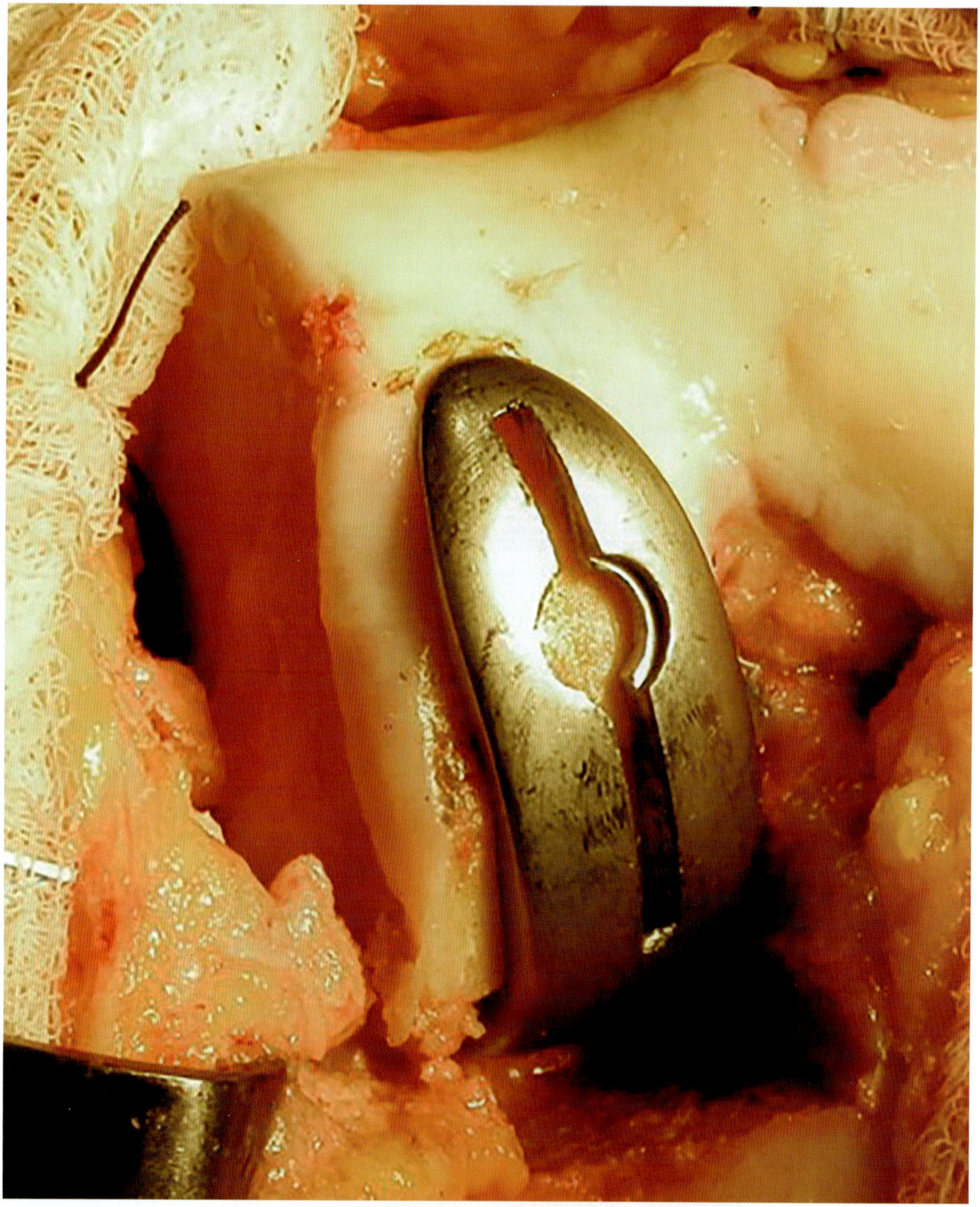

Fig. 8.6 Failure to remove retained distal cartilage from the lateral femoral condyle can lead to prominence of the leading edge of the femoral component with resultant impingement of the patella when the knee is flexed beyond 90 degrees.

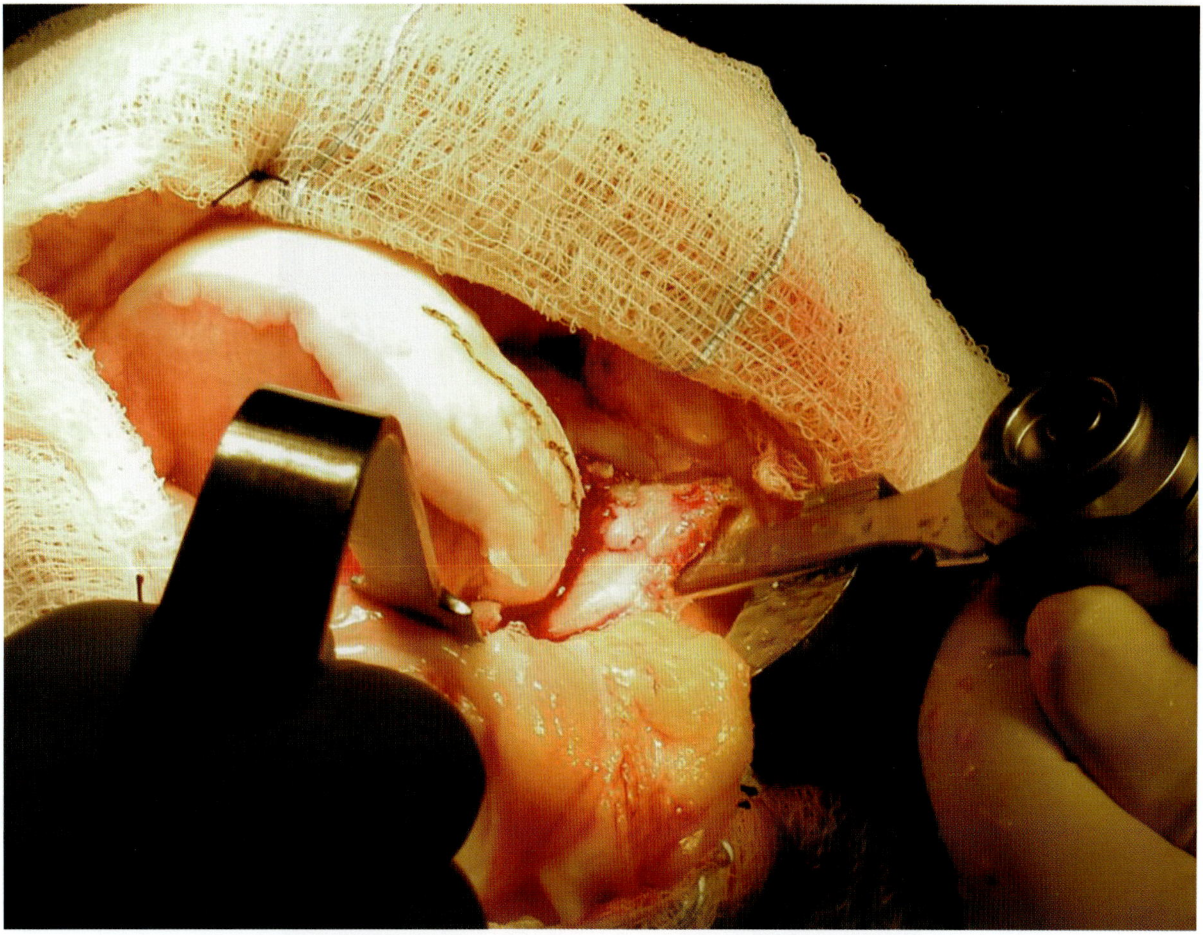

Fig. 8.7 Initial tibial resection in a lateral unicompartmental knee arthroplasty should be conservative.

components to balance the knee that may not be available in any given UKA system.

Over-sizing the anterior–posterior dimension of the femoral component can also lead to patellar impingement and this will require downsizing to avoid the impingement (Fig. 8.8A). When downsizing, it is important to check that adequate metal-to-plastic contact has been maintained when the knee is brought to full extension (Fig. 8.8B).

Optimal femoral component rotation for a lateral arthroplasty is an alignment that is neutral relative to the long axis of the tibial shaft when the knee is flexed 90 degrees (Fig. 8.9). Regarding medial–lateral placement, the surgeon should err toward placing the femoral component laterally (and the tibial component medially) to maximize congruency between the articulating surfaces (Fig. 8.10).

The tendency to place the tibial component too laterally is not an issue with custom components or off-the-shelf tibial components that have different tibial designs for both the medial and lateral tibial components.[6]

Lateral Approach

Most high-volume UKA surgeons actually prefer a lateral approach for lateral UKA and accept the compromises made relative to the medial approach described earlier. A short lateral arthrotomy gives direct exposure to the lateral condyle and plateau.[3,4] The same component positioning principles espoused previously for a medial approach still apply. Recovery will most likely be days faster regarding ability to straight-leg-raise and regain full potential motion.

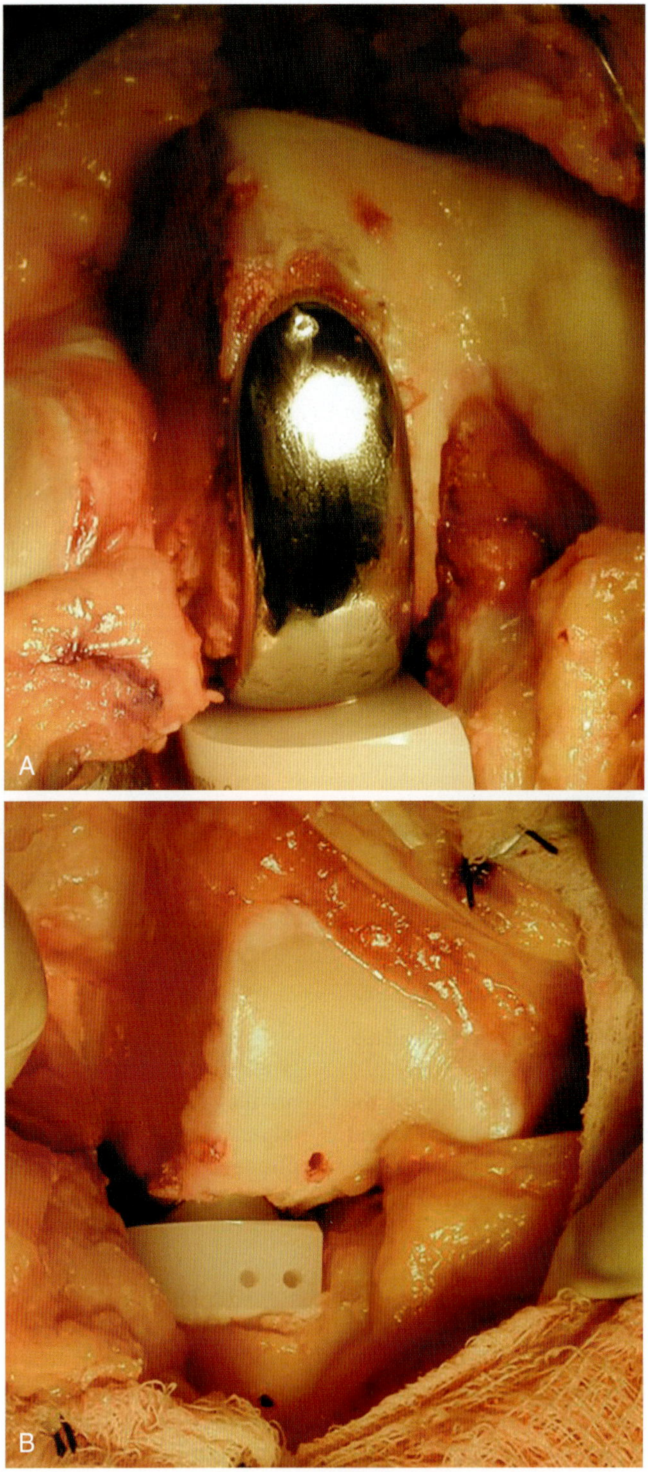

Fig. 8.8 (A) Patellar impingement was resolved in this patient by downsizing the femoral component, allowing recession of its leading edge. (B) After downsizing, adequate metal-to-plastic contact should be maintained in full knee extension.

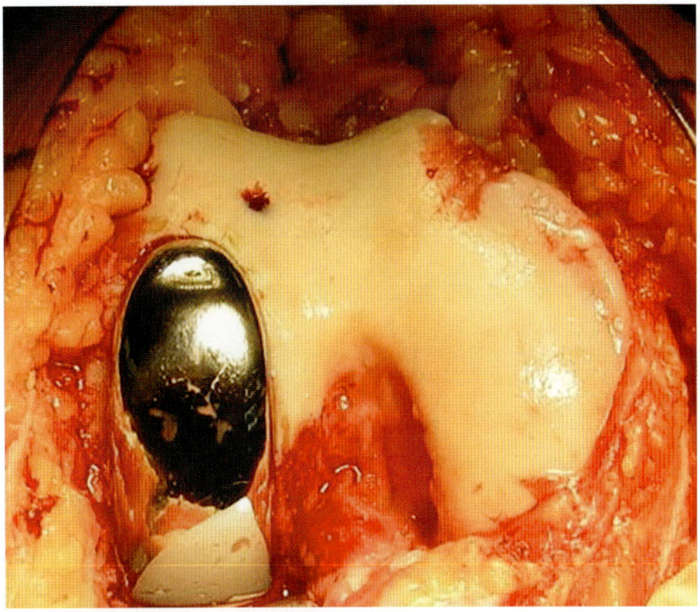

Fig. 8.9 Femoral component rotational orientation should be neutral relative to the long axis of the tibial shaft when the knee is flexed 90 degrees.

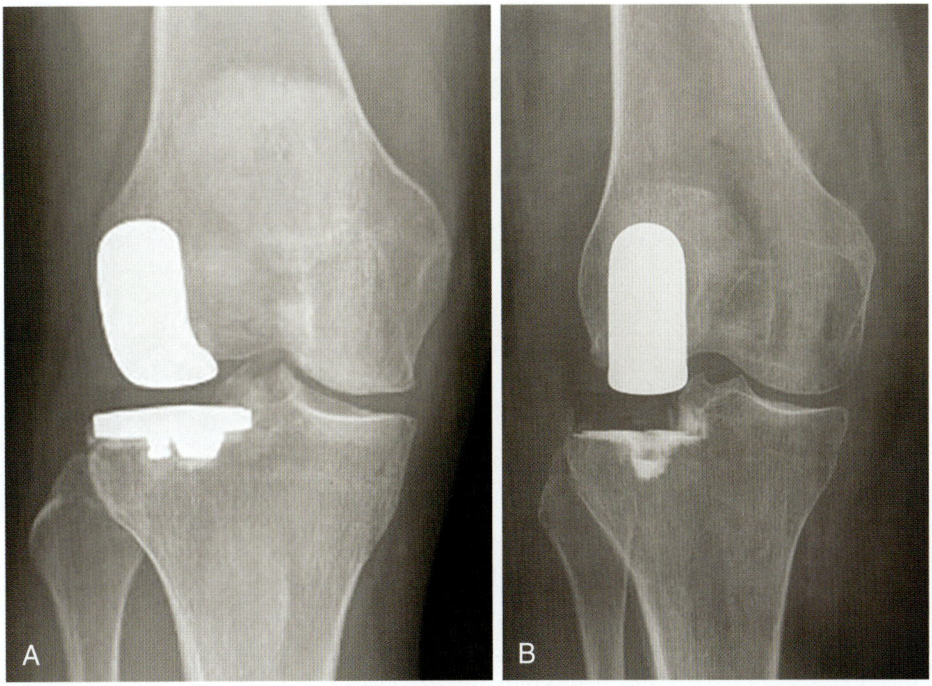

Fig. 8.10 (A) As shown in the radiograph, the femoral component should be placed laterally enough and the tibial component medial enough to create good medial–lateral congruency in the articulation. (B) As shown in this radiograph, when the femoral component is too medial and the tibial component is too lateral, medial–lateral articular incongruency can result.

RECOVERY AND RESULTS

The recovery and results of lateral UKA are similar to those of medial arthroplasty (see Chapter 5). Full restoration of range of motion is common (Fig. 8.11). There are many examples of middle-aged females with lateral arthroplasty returning to vigorous athletic activities (Figs. 8.12 through 8.14). These active patients should understand that they might possibly shorten the longevity of their arthroplasty. But if done well, a lateral UKA is unlikely to compromise any future revision procedure.

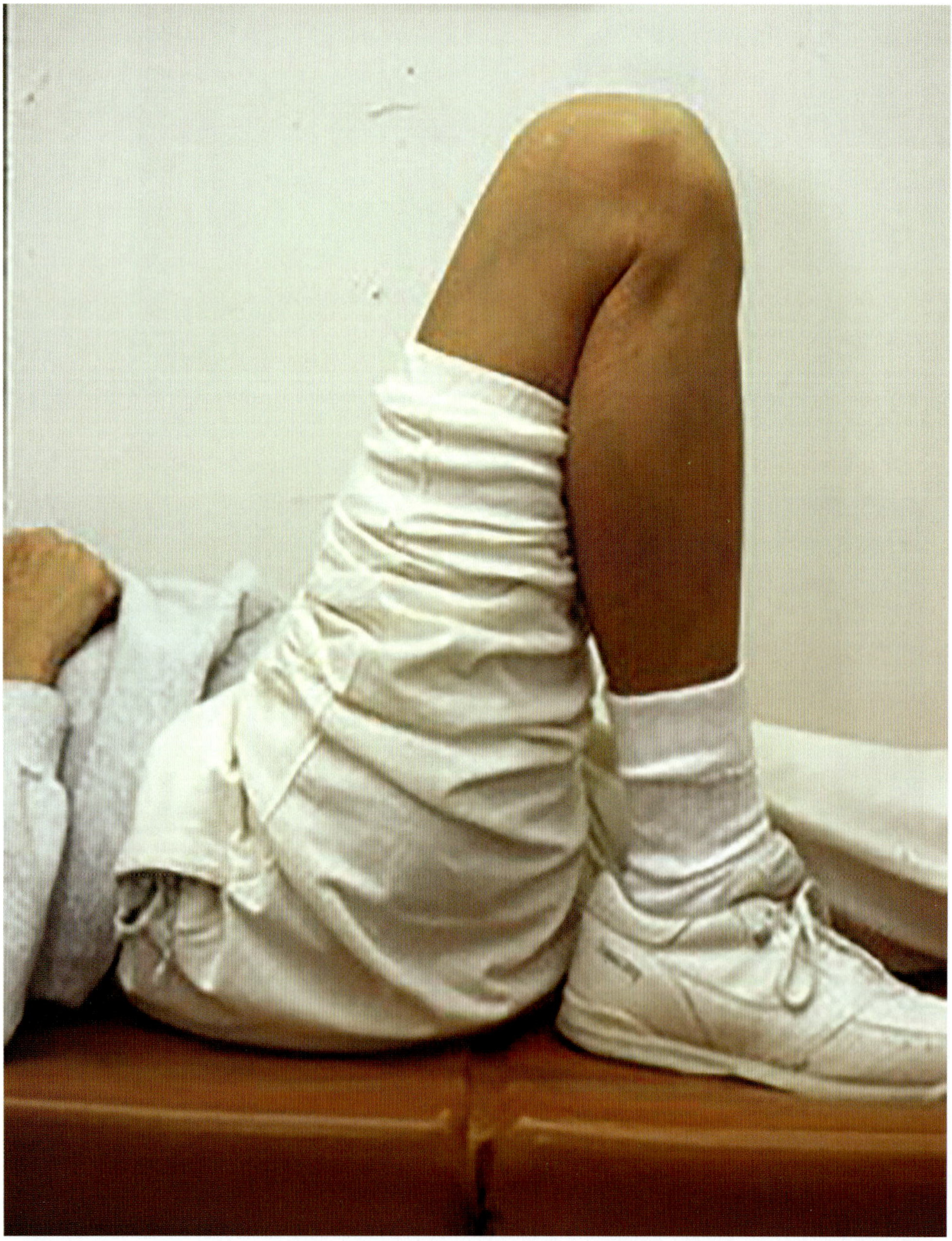

Fig. 8.11 A Lateral Unicompartmental Knee Arthroplasty Is capable of achieving full flexion.

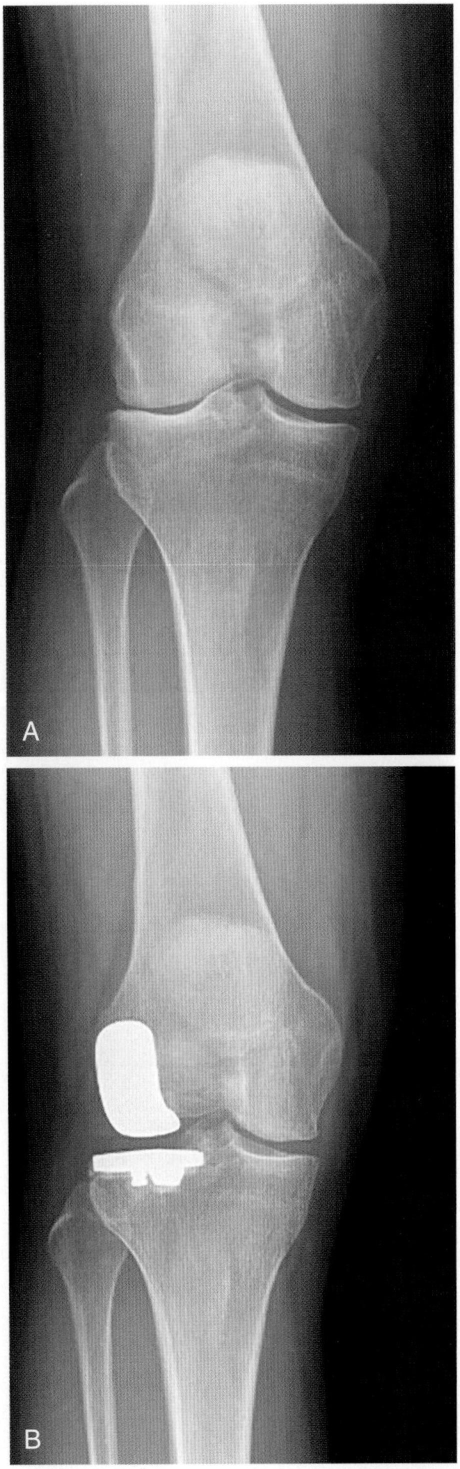

Fig. 8.12 (A) Pre- and (B) postoperative radiographs of a 47-year-old female who returned to skiing black diamond trails after surgery.

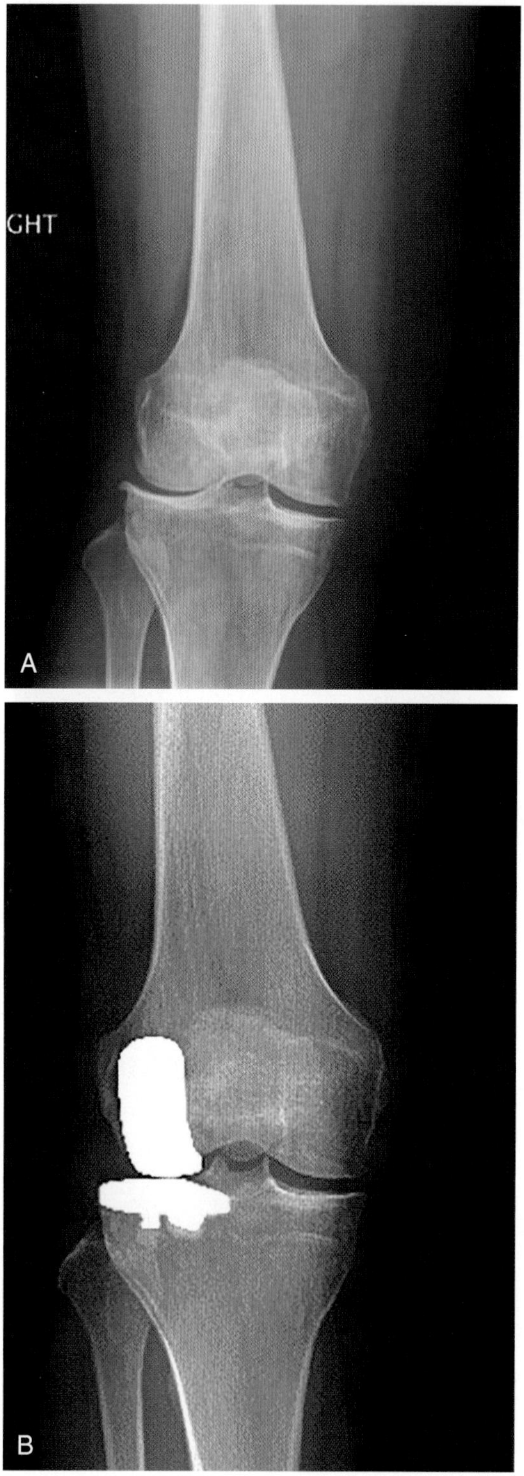

Fig. 8.13 (A) Pre- and (B) postoperative radiographs of a 45-year-old female who returned to competition in national doubles tennis.

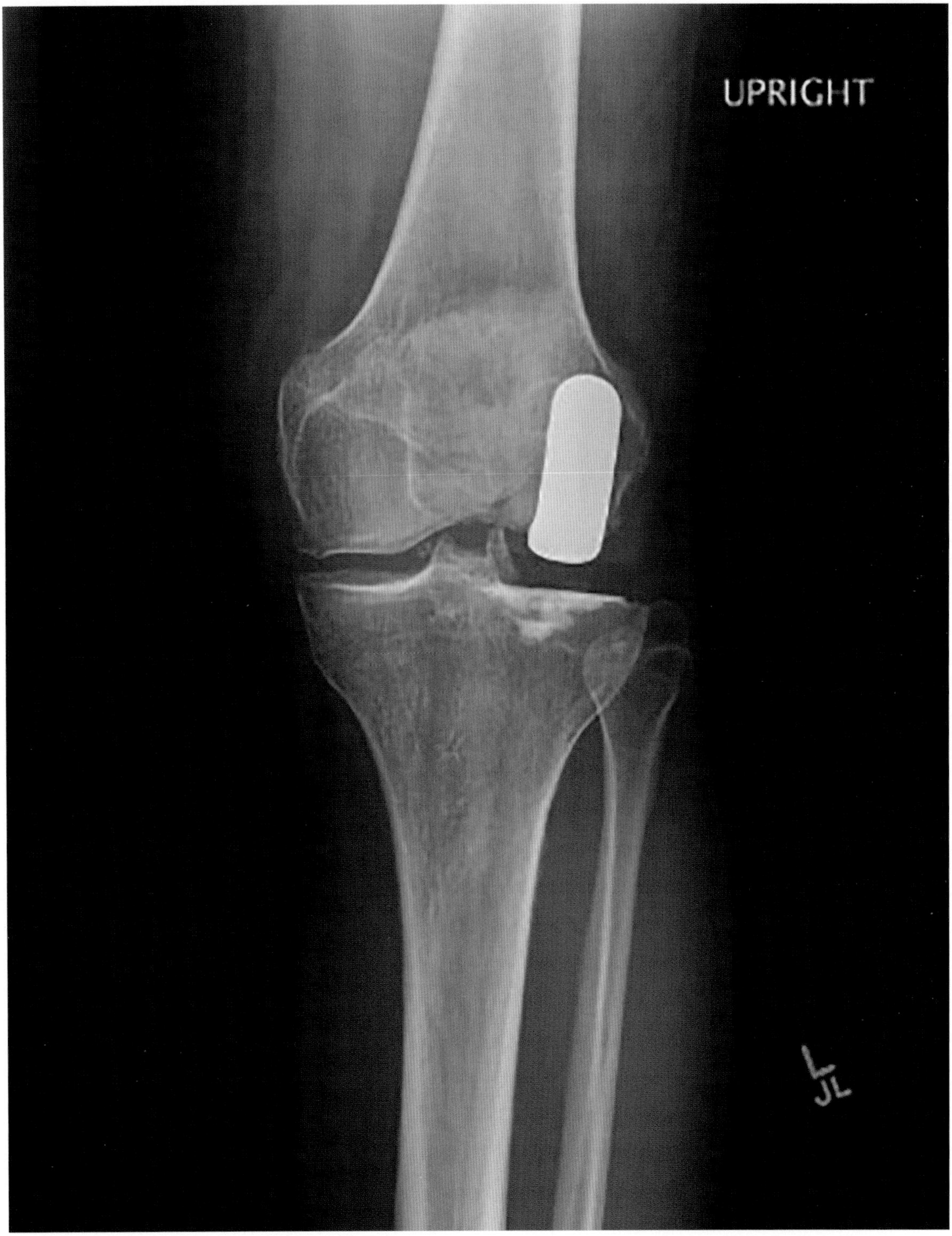

Fig. 8.14 Postoperative radiograph of a 46-year-old female, who was still competing in marathons, triathlons, and international "Iron-man" events at age 55.

REFERENCES

1. White SH, Ludkowski PF, Goodfellow JW. Anteromedial osteoarthritis of the knee. *J Bone Joint Surg Br*. 1991;73: 582–586.
2. Pandit H, Jenkins C, Beard DJ, et al. Mobile bearing dislocation in lateral unicompartmental knee replacement. *Knee*. 2010;17:392–397.
3. Pennington DW, Swienckowski JJ, Lutes WB, Drake GN. Lateral unicompartmental knee arthroplasty: survivorship and technical considerations at an average follow-up of 12.4 years. *J Arthroplasty*. 2006;21:13–17.
4. Ollivier M, Abdel MP, Parrotte S, Argenson JN. Lateral unicondylar arthroplasty: contemporary indications, surgical technique and results. *Int Orthop*. 2014;38: 449–455.
5. Sah AP, Scott RD. Lateral unicompartmental knee arthroplasty through a medial approach: study with an average five-year follow-up. *J Bone Joint Surg Am*. 2007;89:1948–1954.
6. Fitz W, Bliss R, Losina E. Current fit of medial and lateral unicompartmental knee arthroplasty. *Acta Orthop Belg*. 2013;79:191–196.

9

Unicompartmental Knee Arthroplasty in Outliers

Although the "classic" indication for unicompartmental knee arthroplasty (UKA) is isolated end-stage osteoarthritis of the medial or lateral compartment in the elderly patient with an intact anterior cruciate ligament (ACL), other potential indications exist. These "outliers" include selected patients with ACL deficiency. Some patients with the diagnosis of osteonecrosis, as well as middle-aged patients, may be candidates for UKA. Octogenarians are often excluded as candidates, but may also qualify. Finally, UKA may occasionally be indicated after a failed tibial osteotomy or a healed tibial plateau fracture.

THE ACL-DEFICIENT KNEE

A deficient ACL has been said to be a contraindication to UKA based on criteria that were established in the late 1980s.[1] The rationale for this is that a fixed-bearing UKA that imparts little or no anteroposterior (AP) constraint will be unable to restore AP stability to the knee. There are some reports that claim short-term success in these patients if an ACL reconstruction is performed prior to or in conjunction with the arthroplasty.[2,3] Recovery, however, with such a combined procedure(s) can be protracted. The authors, however, have had success performing a fixed-bearing medial UKA in ACL-deficient knees as long as the patient's tibial wear pattern has not progressed posteriorly beyond the mid-third of the tibial plateau and the patient has no subjective complaints of instability. As noted in Chapter 3, the normal tibial wear pattern in medial osteoarthritis is anterior (see Fig. 3.6A). As the disease progresses in an ACL-deficient knee, the wear pattern moves posteriorly (Fig. 9.1). Once it reaches the posterior third of the plateau, stability cannot be restored and long-term success is unlikely. In a mobile-bearing construct, bearing dislocation is also possible.[4]

If a fixed-bearing UKA is performed in an ACL-deficient knee with a mid-third plateau wear pattern, it is important to apply little or no posterior slope to the tibial resection to discourage posterior subluxation, posterior polyethylene wear, and potential tibial loosening.[5] The authors prefer a slope of zero to no more than 3 degrees in these patients (Fig. 9.2).

OSTEONECROSIS

Isolated spontaneous osteonecrosis of the medial femoral condyle with secondary unicompartmental arthritis can be successfully treated with a UKA as long as there is adequate healthy bone remaining after femoral component preparation[6–8] (Fig. 9.3). This can often be predicted preoperatively by obtaining an MRI to assess the surrounding bone structure of the condyle. The status of the remaining bone of the opposite condyle can also be assessed as UKA is contraindicated in multifocal disease such as associated with lupus erythematosus, high-dose steroid usage, and Caisson's disease.

THE MIDDLE-AGED PATIENT

As the initial indications for UKA were focused on the elderly patient, UKA was rarely performed in the middle-aged patient under the age of 60 years. As the mid- and long-term success was established in the elderly, the age criterion was lowered to consider patients in their fourth or fifth decades as a conservative alternative to proximal tibial osteotomy or total knee replacement. Relative to osteotomy, a report by Weale and Newman noted a 10- and 15-year survivorship of UKA of 90% and 88%, respectively, compared with a survivorship of 76% and 65% for high tibial osteotomy (HTO) at similar time intervals.[9] In addition, compared with HTO, a UKA yields

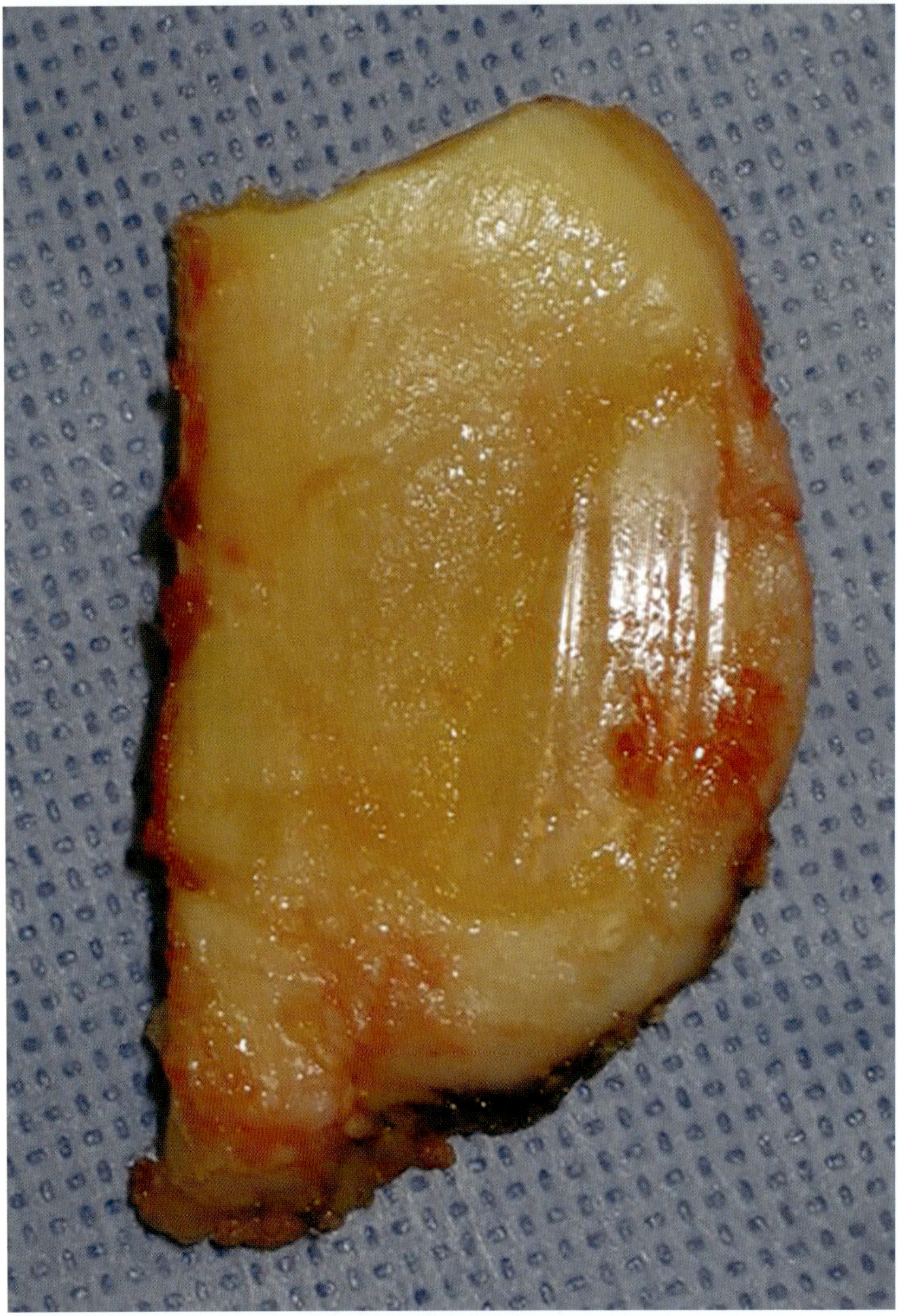

Fig. 9.1 The tibial wear pattern in medial osteoarthritis moves from anterior to posterior when there is ACL deficiency. The central wear pattern shown here allows the patient to remain a candidate for a fixed-bearing UKA. In these cases, little or no posterior slope should be applied to the tibial resection (see text and Fig. 9.2). *ACL,* Anterior cruciate ligament; *UKA,* unicompartmental knee arthroplasty.

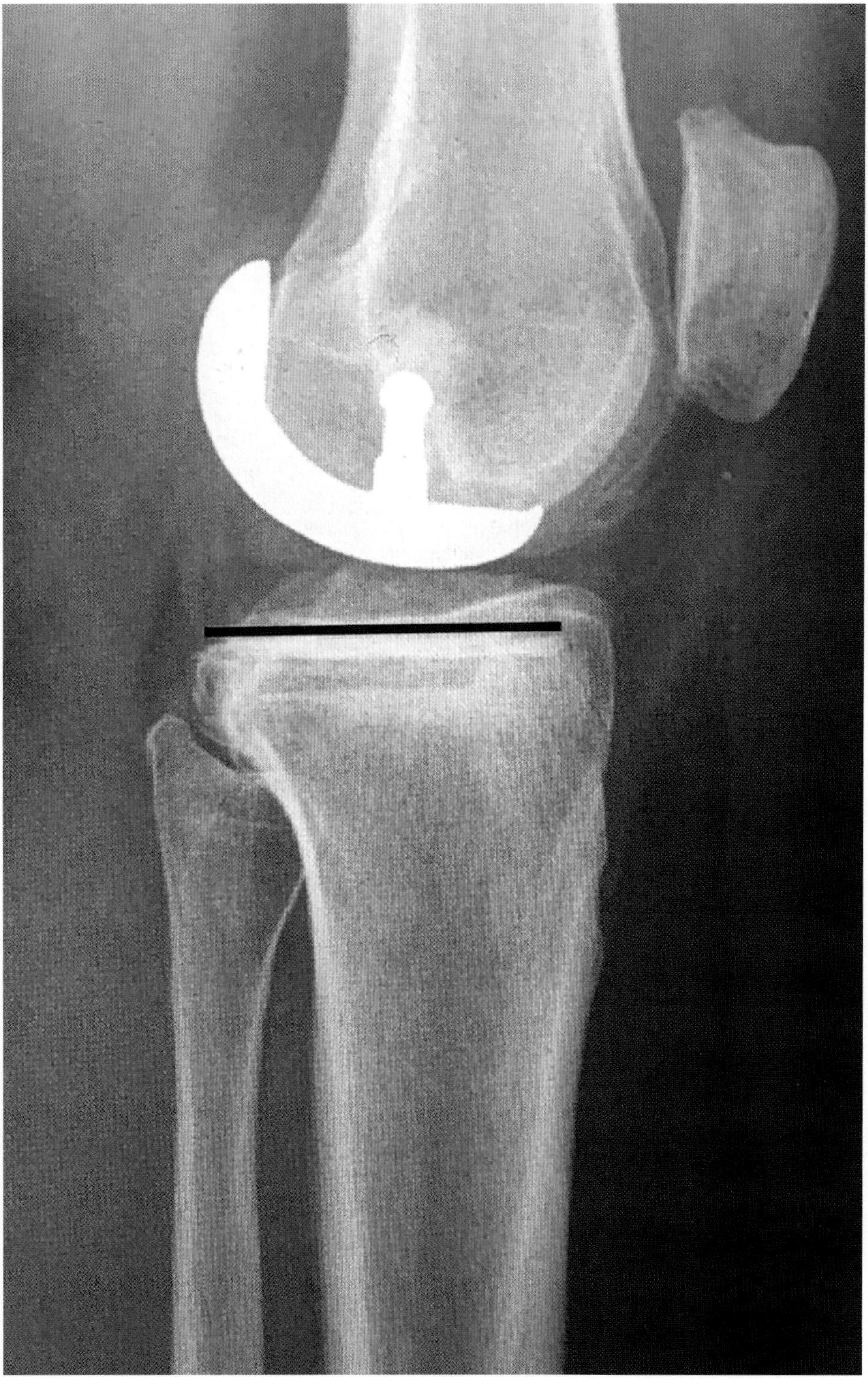

Fig. 9.2 This postoperative lateral radiograph shows that little or no posterior slope has been applied to the tibial resection.

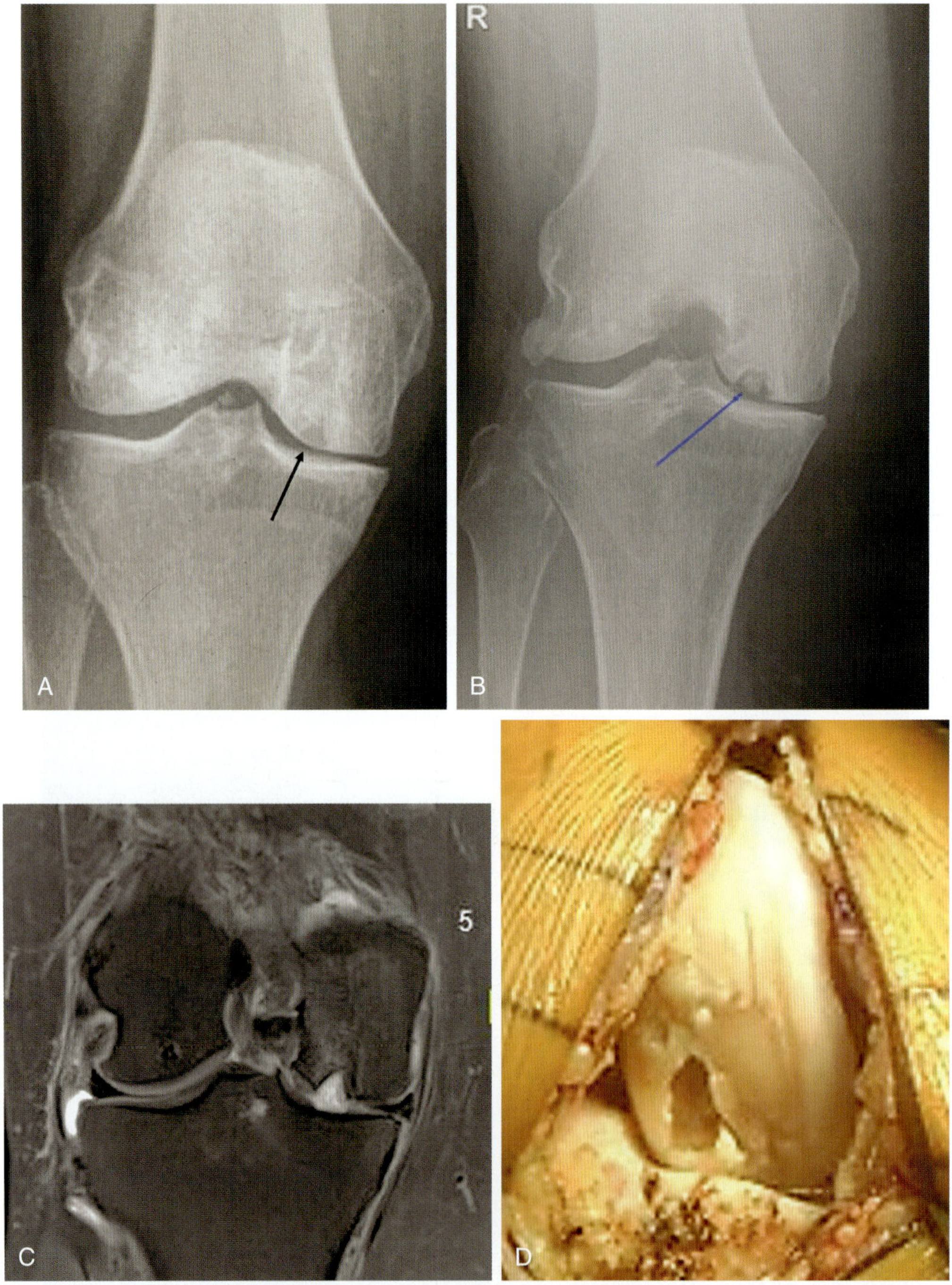

Fig. 9.3 (A) A preoperative standing AP radiograph of a patient with medial weight-bearing pain showing medial joint space narrowing and a suggestion of an area of osteonecrosis involving the medial femoral condyle *(arrow)*. (B) A PA flexed radiograph confirms the area of osteonecrosis *(blue arrow)*. (C) An MRI further defines the area of osteonecrosis and confirms that it is limited to the medial femoral condyle. (D) At surgery, the area of involvement is apparent and after bone preparation there was adequate bone stock to support the cemented femoral component. *AP,* Anteroposterior; *PA,* posteroanterior.

a higher initial success, fewer early complications, and a better cosmetic result. Furthermore, bilateral surgery can be done the same day and conversion, if needed, is easier (see Chapter 10). Advantages of UKA over total knee arthroplasty (TKA) in this middle-aged group of patients include the preservation of both cruciate ligaments, providing more normal knee kinematics and a potentially higher level of performance. Finally, a UKA preserves bone stock compared with a TKA and allows for an easier and less complicated revision should that ever be required (see Chapter 10). Advocates of UKA became even more enthusiastic about performing UKA in younger patients with the advent of minimally invasive UKA (MIU) that allowed a more accelerated recovery with a shortened hospital stay evolving to an outpatient procedure at many centers.[10] The results of UKA in the middle-aged patient have been encouraging in the short- and mid-term.[11–13] The authors' experience has introduced one area of caution regarding the use of UKA in the middle-aged patient. We have observed a higher incidence of UKA failure due to component loosening in middle-aged, mesomorphic male patients (Fig. 9.4). This

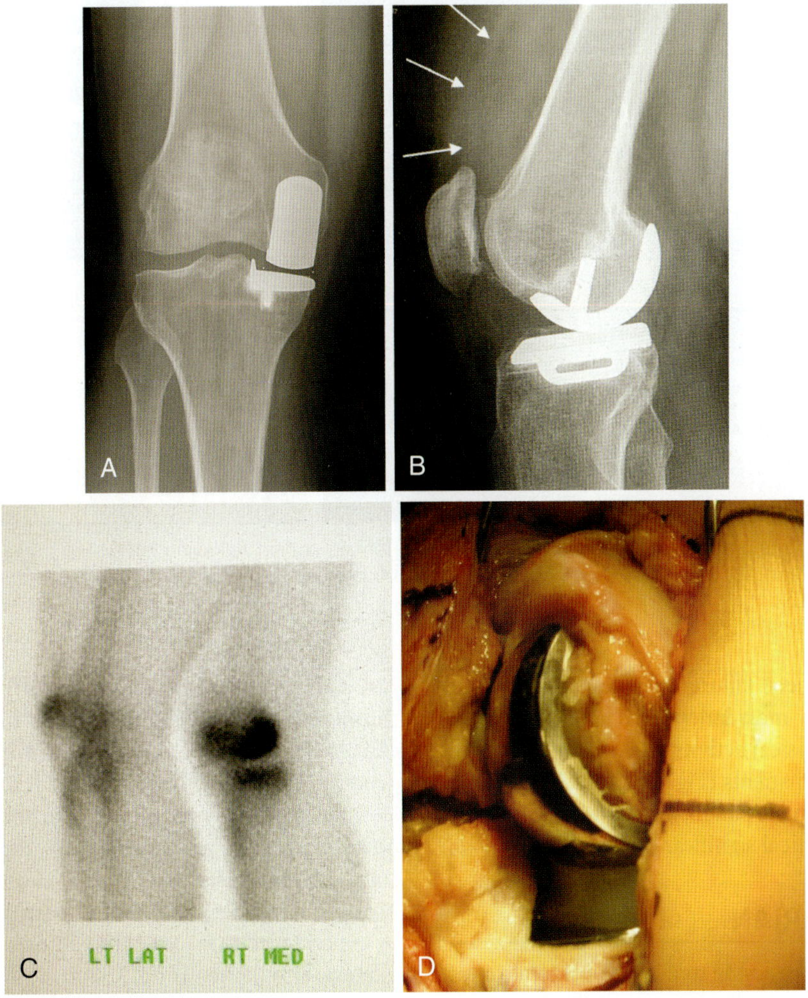

Fig. 9.4 (A) A postoperative radiograph of a 54-year-old mesomorphic male patient showing a well-aligned medial unicompartmental arthroplasty. (B) A lateral radiograph of the same patient 3 years after surgery demonstrates a large knee effusion *(arrows)*. The patient complained of several months of knee swelling and medial weight-bearing pain. There is no obvious evidence of component loosening. (C) A radionucleotide bone scan demonstrates increased activity surrounding the femoral component. (D) At revision surgery, the femoral component was grossly loose. The component used in this system was eventually modified by adding a second fixation lug to enhance fixation.

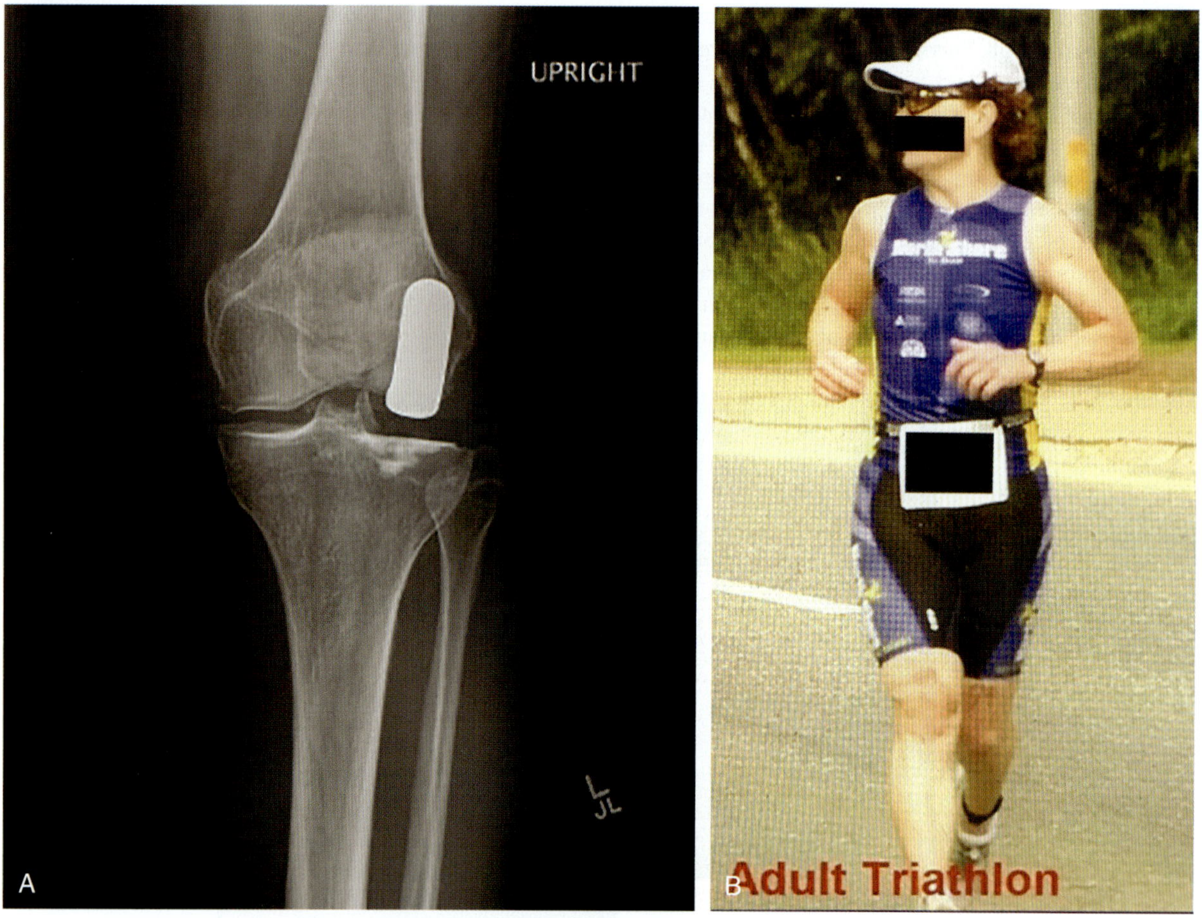

Fig. 9.5 (A) Anteroposterior radiograph of a 46-year-old female patient following lateral unicompartmental knee arthroplasty. (B) Nine years after surgery, the patient continued to participate in "Ironman" and triathlon competitions.

incidence of component failure does not appear to be related to a high body mass index (BMI), but rather to a very high level of physical activity when compared with equally active female patients (Fig. 9.5). Our numbers in this specific group of male patients, however, are not large enough to yield statistical significance.

THE OCTOGENARIAN

The argument could be made to avoid consideration of UKA in an otherwise qualified octogenarian because a TKA will likely last them their projected longevity whereas a UKA has a slightly higher risk of revision. The literature and the authors' experience, however, support consideration of UKA in patients over the age of 80.[14,15] Just as UKA can be described as a first conservative arthroplasty in the younger osteoarthritic patient, a UKA can also be described as the last arthroplasty in the octogenarian. Advantages include a faster recovery, less blood loss, lower risk of complications in the immediate postoperative period, and, usually, less expensive prosthetic components. Survivorship data shows that the UKA prosthesis reliably outlives the patient when implanted by experienced surgeons.[14] In addition, the possibility of bilateral simultaneous UKAs adds to these advantages.[16]

POST–HIGH TIBIAL OSTEOTOMY

Indications for UKA following HTO are infrequent but possible.[17] This infrequency is because a properly executed HTO

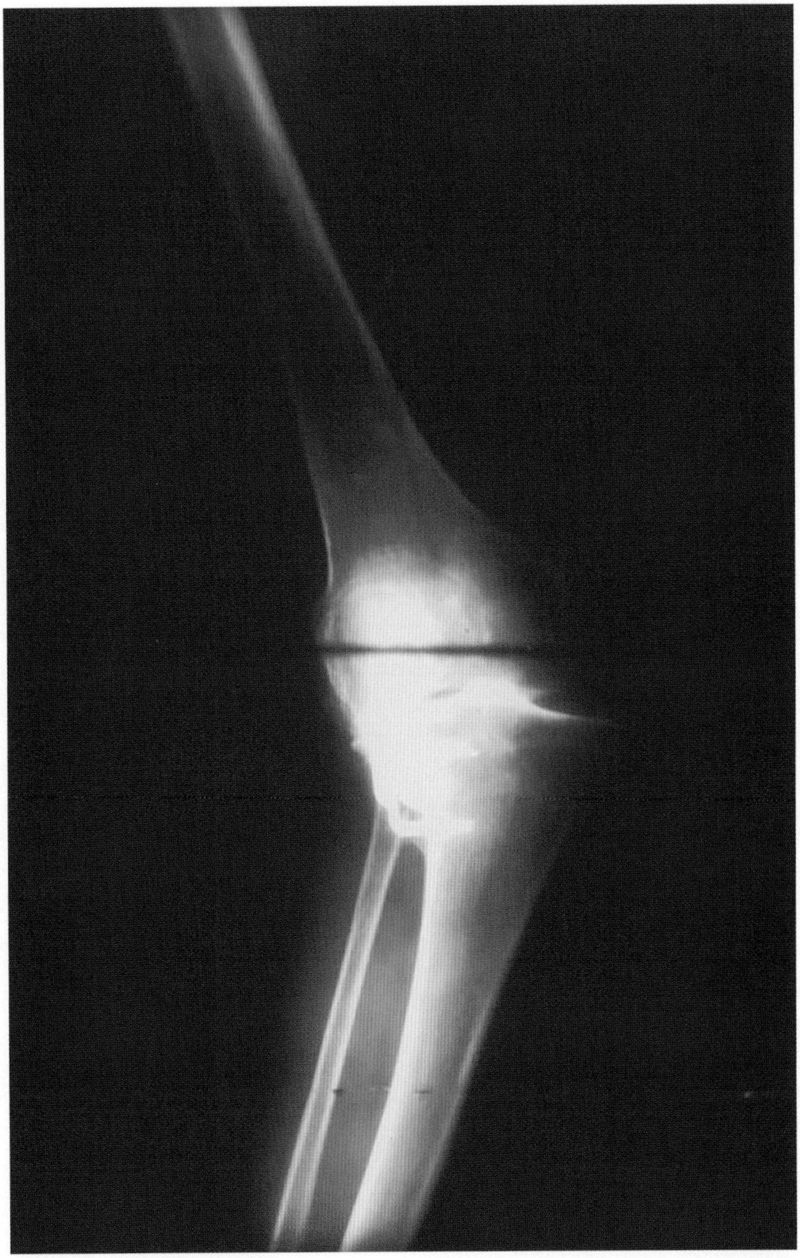

Fig. 9.6 An anteroposterior radiograph of an overcorrected high tibial osteotomy that is not amenable to unicompartmental knee arthroplasty.

converts the mechanical limb alignment into slight valgus. Failure of the osteotomy is often due to secondary degeneration of the opposite compartment creating a situation with bicompartmental involvement. Failure due to overcorrection will possibly be a complicated TKA (Fig. 9.6). In addition, a medial UKA performed after a valgus osteotomy will tend to increase the valgus limb alignment when the medial compartment is replaced and the medial ligaments are brought into proper tension (Fig. 9.7). The most appropriate post-HTO candidate for a UKA is one whose

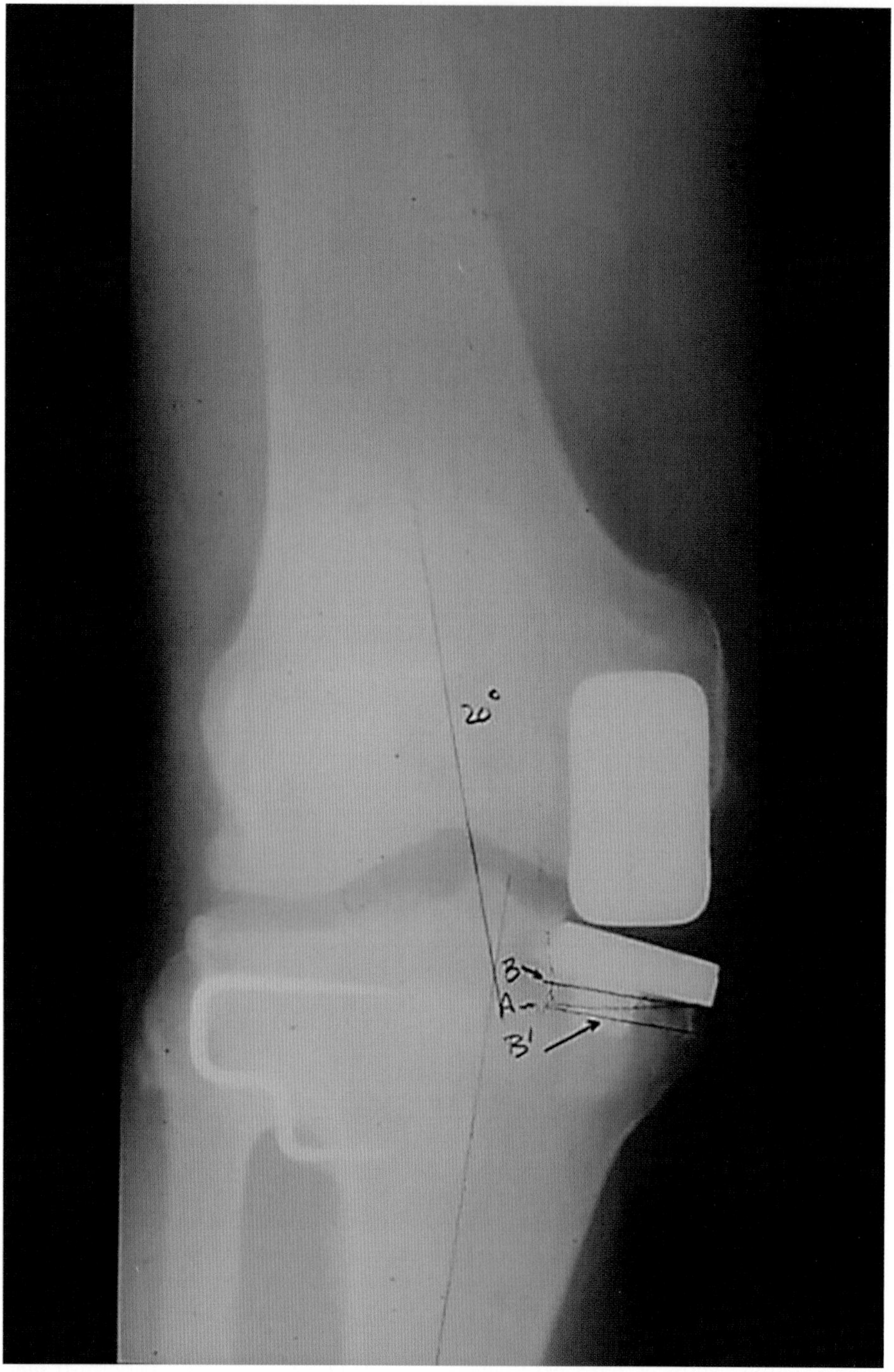

Fig. 9.7 This poorly performed unicompartmental knee arthroplasty (UKA) shows an unsuccessful attempt to treat a healed valgus tibial osteotomy with a UKA. The alignment is overcorrected and the components lack congruency.

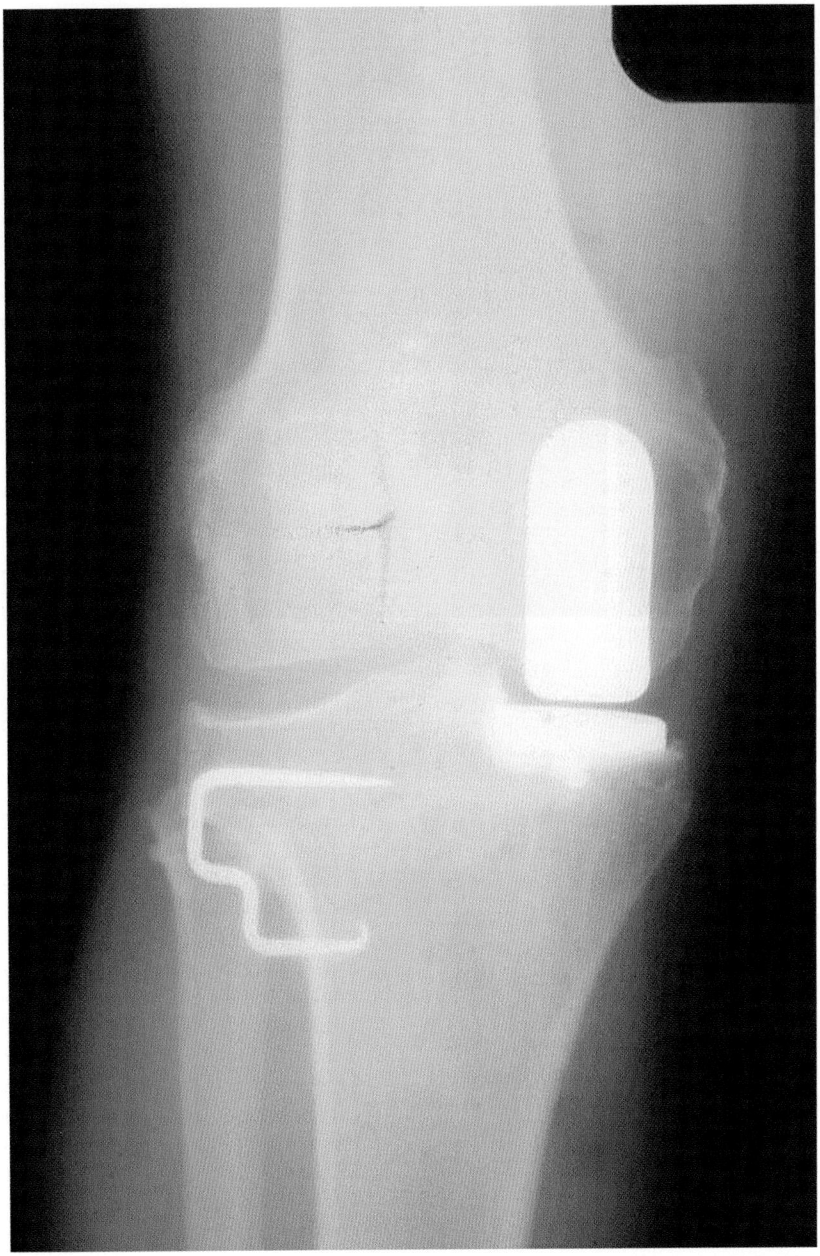

Fig. 9.8 This postoperative radiograph demonstrates a unicompartmental knee arthroplasty that was performed after an undercorrected high tibial osteotomy and shows satisfactory postoperative knee alignment.

alignment has been undercorrected with failure due to persistent medial pain while the other compartments remain normal. A final advantage of UKA to salvage a failed HTO is the possibility to retain the hardware used to secure the osteotomy (Fig. 9.8).

POST–TIBIAL PLATEAU FRACTURE

On rare occasions, UKA may be indicated to replace a single compartment after a healed tibial plateau fracture. There is no literature reporting a series of such

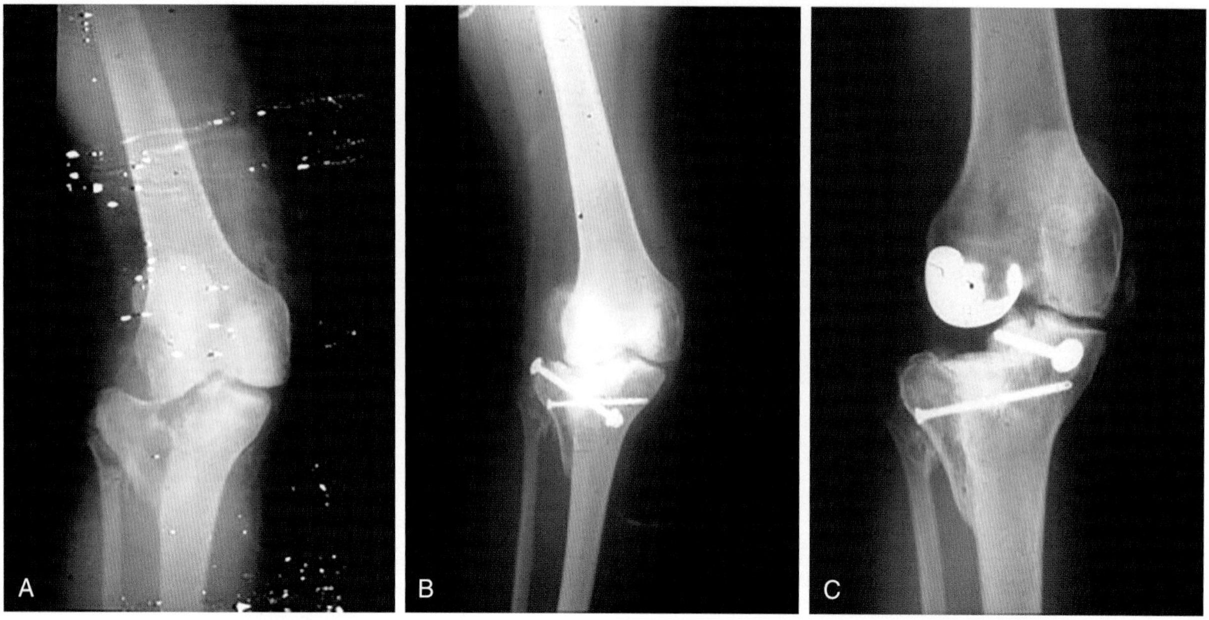

Fig. 9.9 (A) A radiograph showing a severe comminuted tibial fracture involving the lateral tibial plateau. (B) After open reduction and internal fixation, the fracture healed but the patient had a painful ankylosed knee with only 5 degrees of knee motion. (C) Twenty years after reconstruction with a lateral unicompartmental knee arthroplasty combined with a V-Y quadricepsplasty, the patient was pain free and maintained 90 degrees of knee flexion.

patients. To be such a candidate, the patient would have to have healed their fracture and have sufficient bone stock to support the tibial component. The senior author has experience with several such patients, the most extreme of whom is shown in Fig. 9.9. This patient presented with an ankylosed knee with 10 degrees of motion after she had healed her open reduction and internal fixation. Twenty years after her UKA combined with a V-Y quadriceps lengthening,[18] she was pain free and maintaining 90 degrees of knee flexion. Possible future conversion to a TKA was not compromised by her UKA procedure.

REFERENCES

1. Kozinn SC, Scott RD. Unicondylar knee arthroplasty: current concepts review. *J Bone Joint Surg Am.* 1989;71:145–150.
2. Pandit H, Beard DJ, Jenkins C, et al. Combined anterior cruciate reconstruction and Oxford unicompartmental knee arthroplasty. *J Bone Joint Surg Br.* 2006;88(7):887–892.
3. Zumbrunn T, Schütz P, von Knoch F, Preiss S, List R, Ferguson SJ. Medial unicompartmental knee arthroplasty in ACL-deficient knees is a viable treatment option: in vivo kinematic evaluation using a moving fluoroscope. *Knee Surg Sports Traumatol Arthrosc.* 2020;28(6):1765–1773.
4. Callaghan JJ. Mobile-bearing knee replacement: clinical results: a review of the literature. *Clin Orthop Relat Res.* 2001;(392):221–225.
5. Hernigou P, Deschamps G. Posterior slope of the tibial implant and the outcome of unicompartmental knee arthroplasty. *J Bone Joint Surg Am.* 2004;86(3):506–511.
6. Kaneko T, Kono N, Sunakawa T, Okuno Y, Ikegami H, Musha Y. Reliable patient-reported outcome measure and survivorship of UKA for primary spontaneous osteonecrosis. *Eur J Orthop Surg Traumatol.* 2019;29(1):119–124.
7. Ollivier M, Jacquet C, Lucet A, Parratte S, Argenson JN. Long-term results of medial unicompartmental knee arthroplasty for knee avascular necrosis. *J Arthroplasty.* 2019;34(3):465–468.
8. Chalmers BP, Mehrotra KG, Sierra RJ, Pagnano MW, Taunton MJ, Abdel MP. Reliable outcomes and survivorship of unicompartmental knee arthroplasty for isolated compartment osteonecrosis. *Bone Joint J.* 2018;100-B(4):450–454.
9. Weale AE, Newman JH. Unicompartmental arthroplasty and high tibial osteotomy for osteoarthrosis of the knee. A comparative study with a 12- to 17-year follow-up period. *Clin Orthop Relat Res.* 1994;(302):134–137.

10. Repicci JA, Hartman JF. Minimally invasive unicondylar knee arthroplasty for the treatment of unicompartmental osteoarthritis: an outpatient arthritic bypass procedure. *Orthop Clin North Am*. 2004;35:201–216.
11. Heyse TJ, Khefacha A, Peersman G, Cartier P. Survivorship of UKA in the middle-aged. *Knee*. 2012;19(5):585–591.
12. Kim KT, Lee S, Lee JS, Kang MS, Koo KH. Long-term clinical results of unicompartmental knee arthroplasty in patients younger than 60 years of age: minimum 10-year follow-up. *Knee Surg Relat Res*. 2018;30(1):28–33.
13. Lee M, Chen J, Shi Lu C, Lo NN, Yeo SJ. No differences in outcomes scores or survivorship of unicompartmental knee arthroplasty between patients younger or older than 55 years of age at minimum 10-year followup. *Clin Orthop Relat Res*. 2019;477(6):1434–1446.
14. Sah AP, Springer BD, Scott RD. Unicompartmental knee arthroplasty in octogenarians: survival longer than the patient. *Clin Orthop*. 2006;4:107–112.
15. Ode Q, Gaillard R, Batailler C, et al. Fewer complications after UKA than TKA in patients over 85 years of age: a case-control study. *Orthop Traumatol Surg Res*. 2018;104(7):955–959.
16. Cahill CW, Schwarzkopf R, Sinha S, Scott RD. Simultaneous bilateral knee arthroplasty in octogenarians: can it be safe and effective? *J Arthroplasty*. 2014;29(5): 998–1000.
17. Valenzuela GA, Jacobson NA, Buzas D, Koreckij TD, Valenzuela RG, Teitge RA. Unicompartmental knee replacement after high tibial osteotomy: invalidating a contraindication. *Bone Joint J*. 2013;95-B(10): 1348–1353.
18. Scott RD, Siliski JM. The use of a modified V-Y quadricepsplasty during total knee replacement to gain exposure and improve flexion in the ankylosed knee. *Orthopedics*. 1986;8:45–48.

10

Revision of Failed Unicompartmental Knee Arthroplasty

One of the principal advantages of unicompartmental knee arthroplasty (UKA) is its conservative nature. Ideally, after a UKA, any future revision can be carried out with the use of primary total knee arthroplasty (TKA) components and the result can be comparable to a primary arthroplasty. Initial experience from the 1980s indicated that this might not be the case.[1] As experience with primary UKA was gained, however, subsequent reports confirmed its conservative nature.[2–5]

TIBIAL REVISION

For a UKA to be conservative, it is important that surgeons follow the basic principle of performing a minimal initial tibial resection[6] (see Chapter 6). By doing so, tibial augmentation methods such as modular wedges will rarely be required (Fig. 10.1). When initial tibial resection has been excessive (Fig. 10.2), augmentation methods and extended tibial stems will be required.

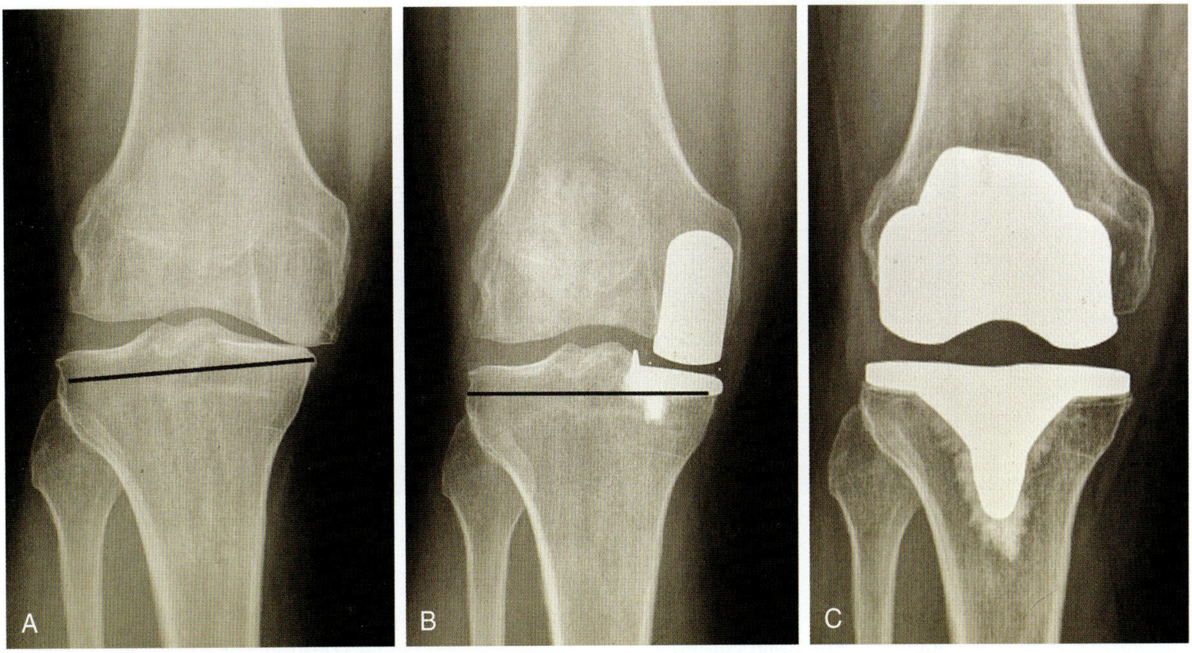

Fig. 10.1 (A) An anteroposterior (AP) radiograph prior to a unicompartmental knee arthroplasty showing a planned medial tibial resection based on a conservative lateral resection for a total knee arthroplasty. (B) A postoperative radiograph in the same patient showing the proper execution of the conservative preoperative plan. (C) An AP radiograph in the same patient 3 years later after revision for femoral component loosening. Standard components were utilized without the need for any augmentation method.

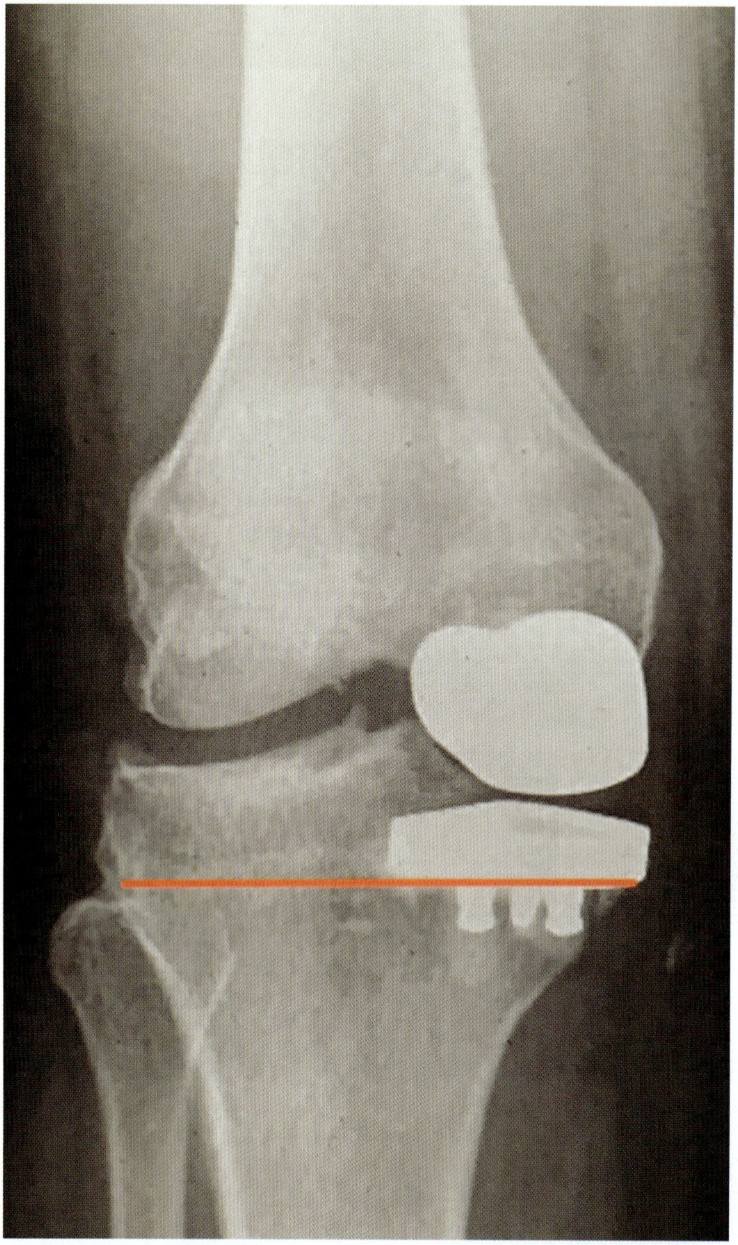

Fig. 10.2 A postoperative anteroposterior radiograph of a unicompartmental knee arthroplasty exhibiting excessive tibial resection that will compromise any future revision.

Loss of tibial bone stock following a medial UKA can also be due to subsidence of the tibial component, although osteolysis compromising tibial bone stock is rare. An example of this is shown in Fig. 10.3. In this case, the tibial component had slowly subsided over a 20-year period. The resultant defect was significant, but was mostly contained by cortical bone and could be treated with a tibial component with a 30-mm stem extension and the use of local autogenous bone graft harvested from standard total knee bone resections.

After failed lateral UKA, loss of tibial bone stock is also rarely a problem (Fig. 10.4). This is most likely because

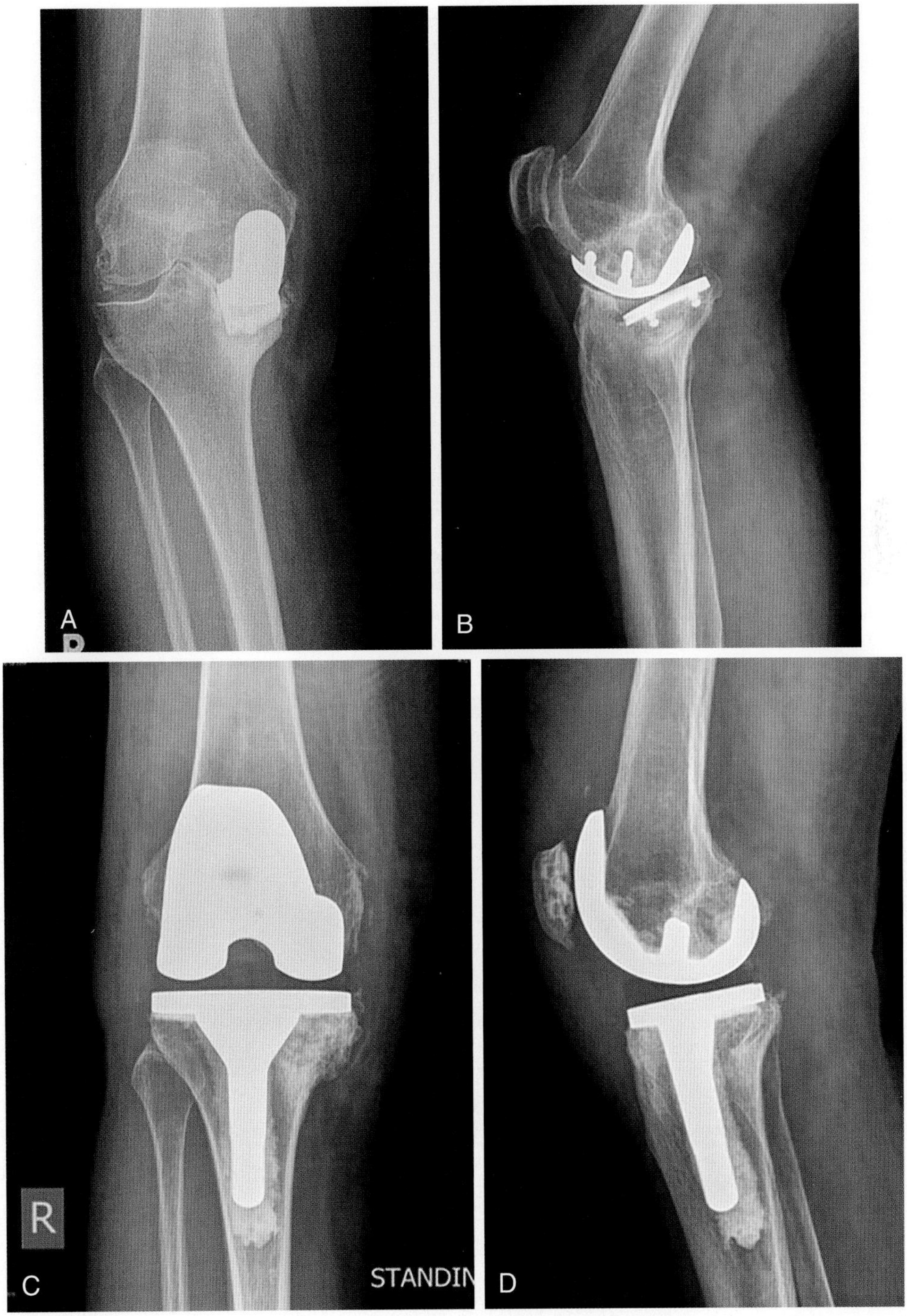

Fig. 10.3 (A and B) An anteroposterior (AP) and lateral radiograph showing a loose subsided tibial component 20 years after the index unicompartmental knee arthroplasty. (C and D) An immediate postoperative AP and lateral radiograph following revision with a standard femoral component, an extended-stemmed tibial component, and the use of autologous bone graft to fill the contained defect (harvested from the femoral and tibial bone resections).

Continued

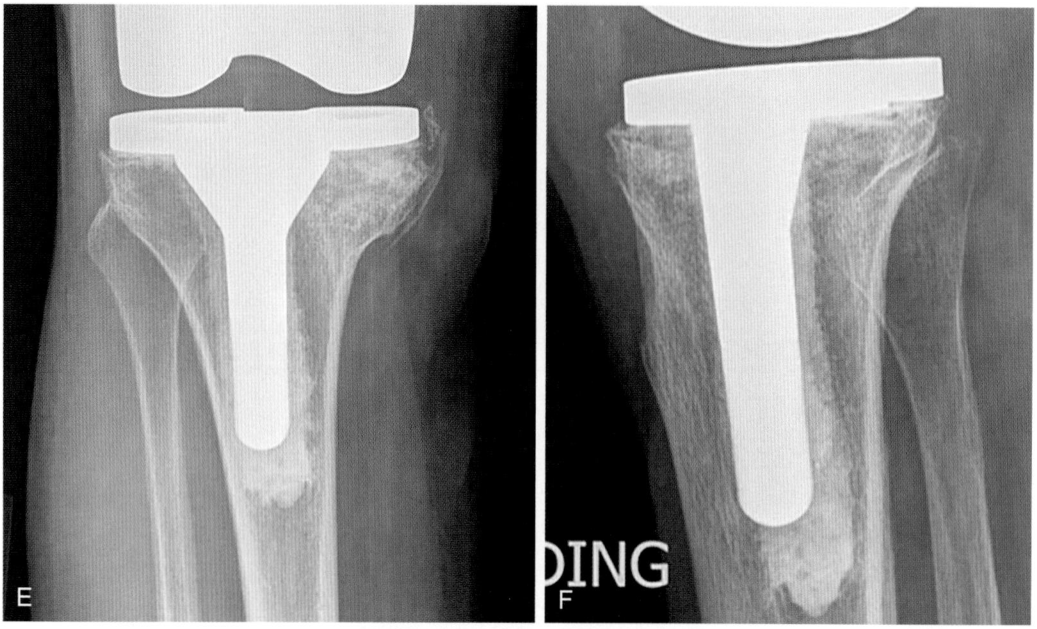

Fig. 10.3, cont'd (E and F) A 1-year follow-up AP and lateral radiograph showing apparent incorporation of the bone graft without component subsidence. The patient was asymptomatic at 9-year follow-up.

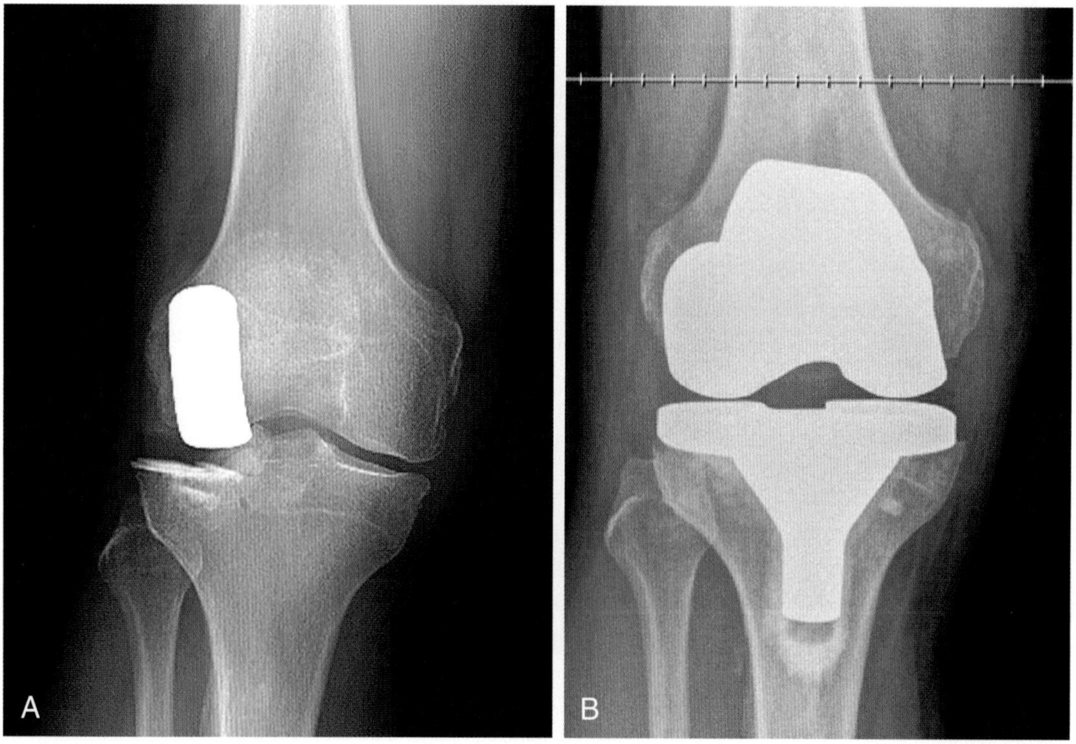

Fig. 10.4 (A) An anteroposterior radiograph showing a failed lateral unicompartmental knee arthroplasty. (B) A postoperative radiograph of the same patient following revision using standard components.

tibial bone preparation for lateral UKA is intrinsically conservative (see Chapter 8).

FEMORAL REVISION

On the femoral side, UKA revision is rarely compromised by the presence of a previously implanted femoral component unless the femoral fixation method involved the use of deeply penetrating fins or lugs that were utilized occasionally in early designs (Fig. 10.5). In these cases, surgeons must be careful in the removal of such components and be prepared for the potential need for bone graft, augmentation wedges, and stemmed femoral components. Almost all contemporary UKA femoral components are conservative in nature in their fixation method, thickness of the metallic femoral condyle, and requirement for bone resection during implantation (Fig. 10.6). After their removal, sufficient femoral bone stock is still available even if the surgeon advocates cementless fixation (Figs. 10.7 and 10.8).

After failed lateral UKA, there may be some slight deficiency of the lateral posterior femoral condyle following component removal. This may be due to the intrinsic relative hypoplasia of the lateral condyle in osteoarthritic valgus knees or due to some intentional slight posterior condylar overresection to relieve tightness in flexion at the time of the initial arthroplasty. This deficiency can be filled with cement if very minor or with a posterior augment if required. A third potential solution is the use of a high flexion femoral component available in some systems. These components are manufactured with a thicker-than-normal posterior metallic condyle to allow greater metal-to-plastic contact with knee flexion angles up to 150 degrees (Fig. 10.9).

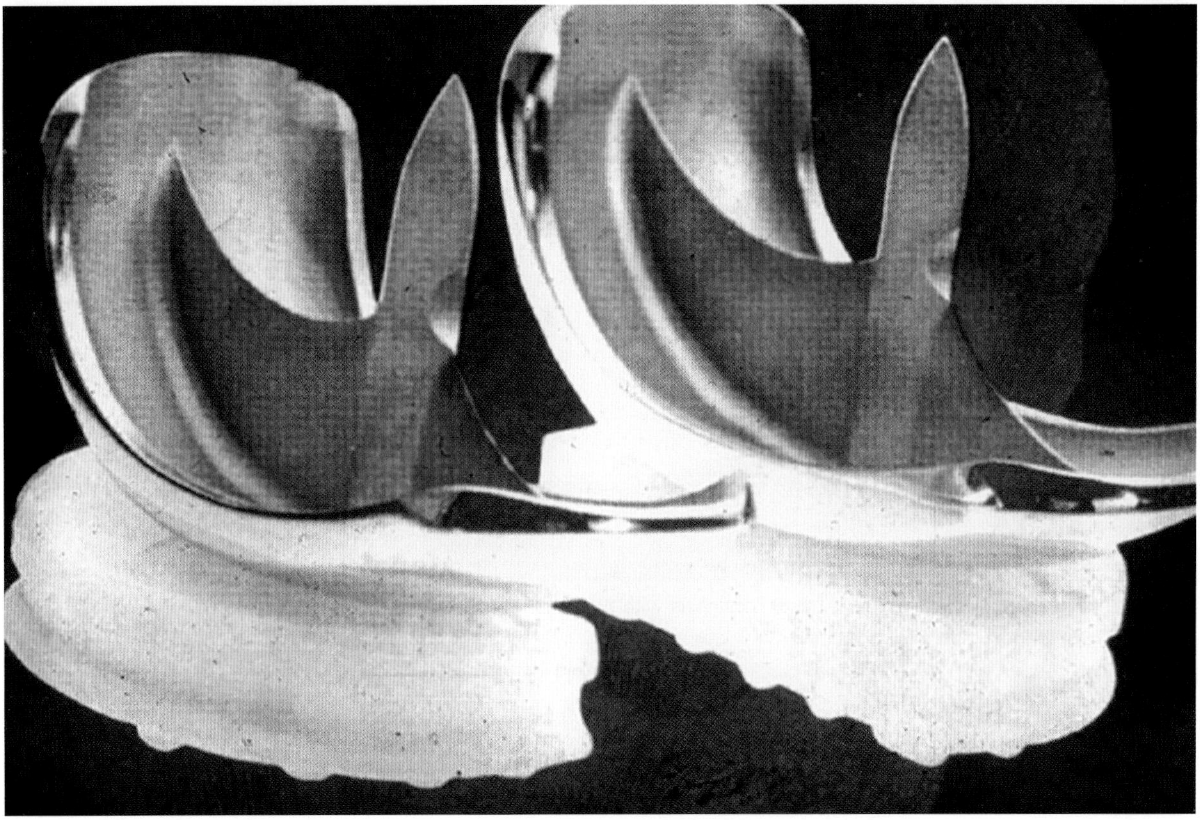

Fig. 10.5 An early generation unicompartmental knee arthroplasty femoral prosthesis with a lug and fin that deeply penetrated the femoral condyle and often led to loss of femoral bone stock upon removal.

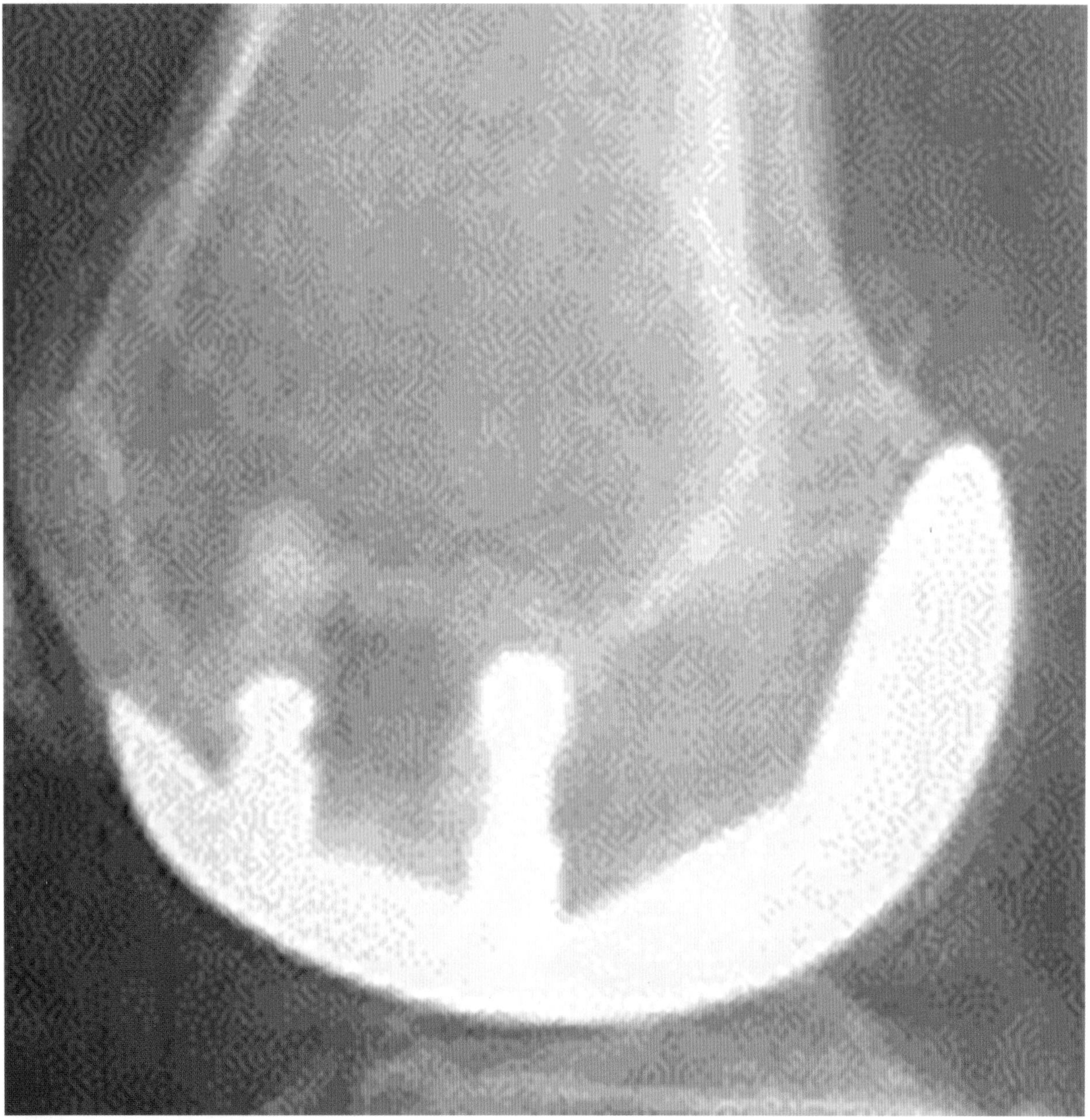

Fig. 10.6 A contemporary femoral prosthesis with two lugs for fixation that is unlikely to compromise bone stock upon removal.

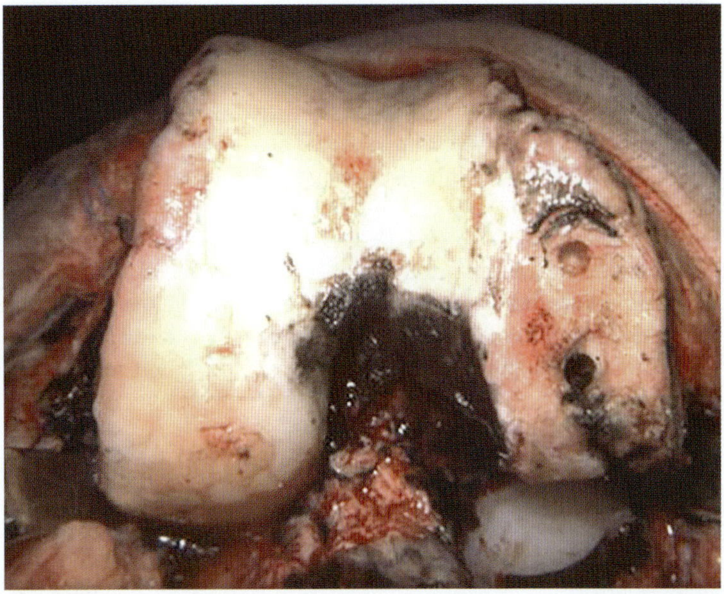

Fig. 10.7 An intraoperative photograph showing no compromise of femoral bone stock after the removal of a contemporary style two-lugged femoral component.

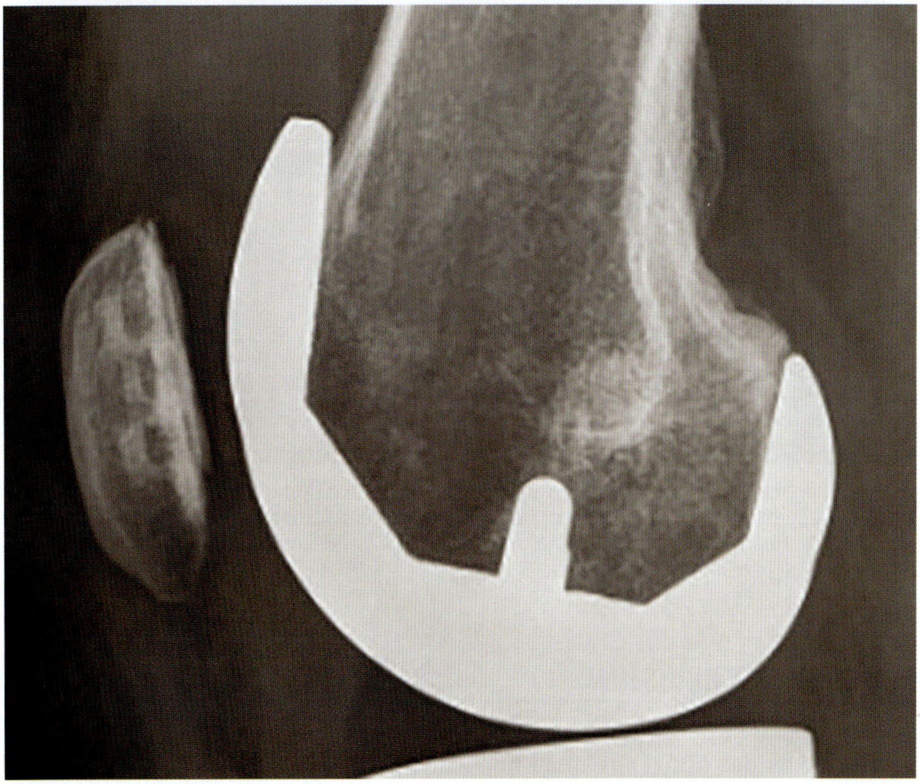

Fig. 10.8 A lateral radiograph of the femur after revision of a failed unicompartmental knee arthroplasty using a cementless femoral component.

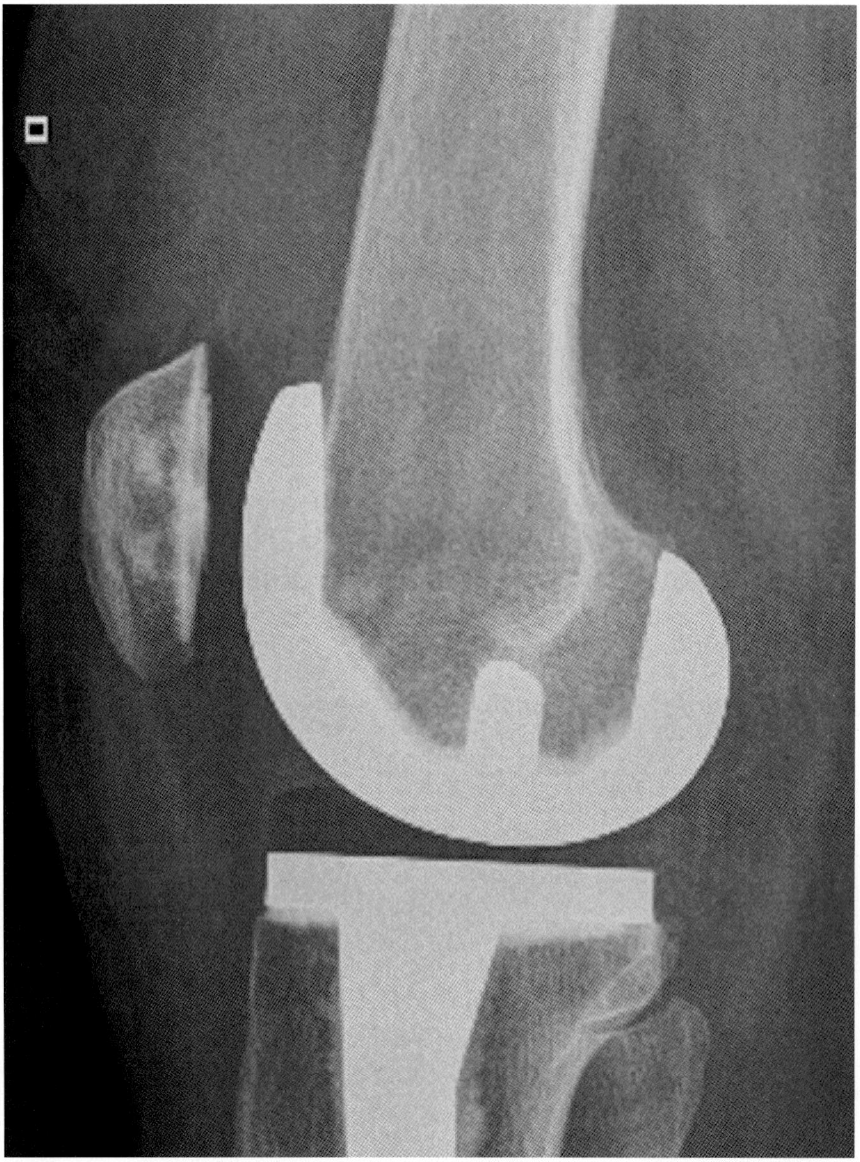

Fig. 10.9 A lateral radiograph of a "high-flex" femoral component demonstrating posterior femoral condyles that are approximately 2 mm thicker than those on a standard femoral component from the same system. These components can be utilized in the revision of a failed lateral unicompartmental knee arthroplasty where there is minor posterior condylar deficiency.

ISOLATED COMPONENT REVISION

If a UKA fails because of polyethylene wear in a modular tibial component or residual instability in an undercorrected arthroplasty, isolated insert revision can be considered (Fig. 10.10). These types of cases are relatively rare and there are no long-term reports of series consisting of isolated component revision for these issues. Isolated bearing exchange for mobile-bearing dislocation has been reported with some short-term success, but large series with long-term results are not available.[7–9]

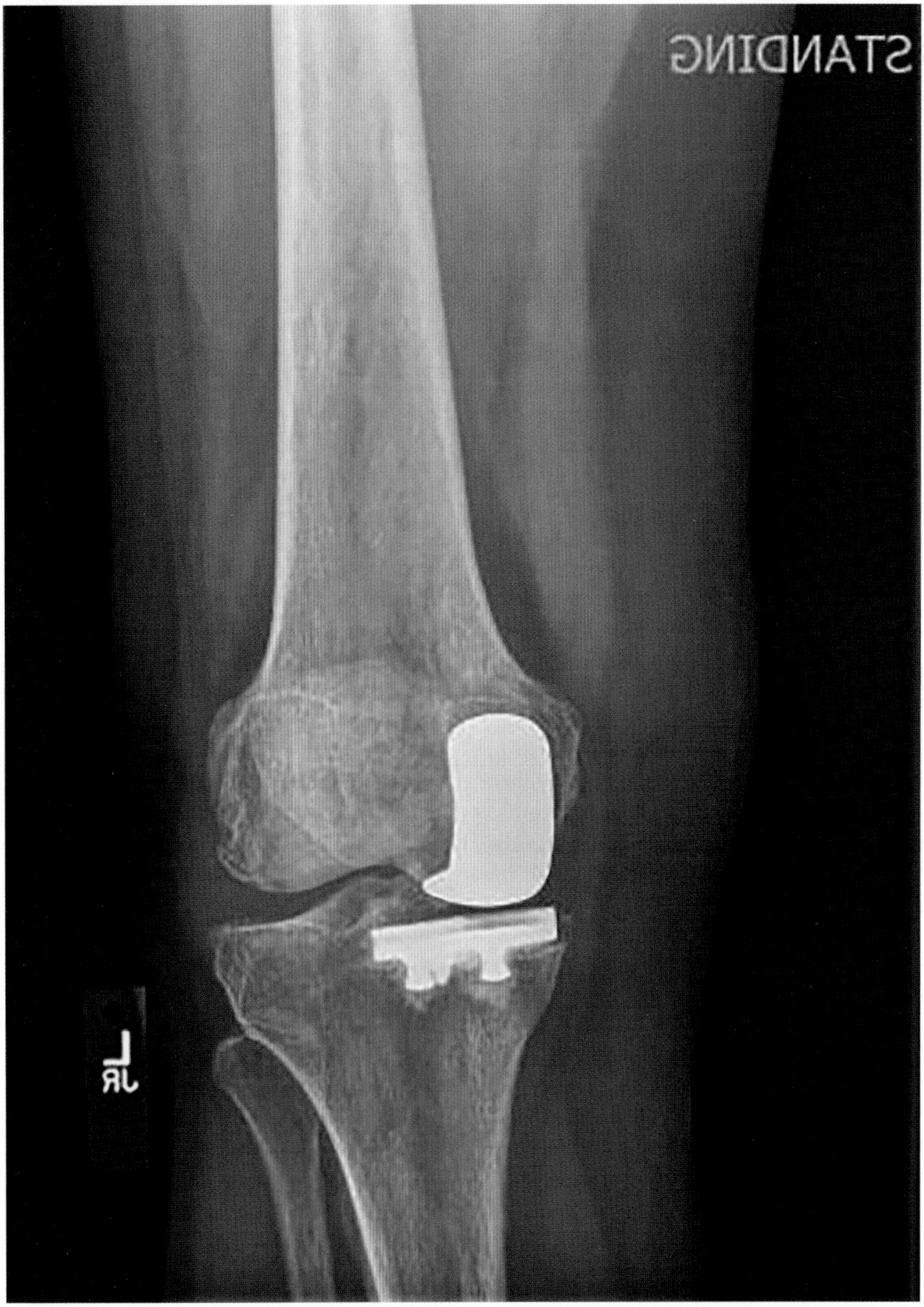

Fig. 10.10 An anteroposterior radiograph of an undercorrected unicompartmental knee arthroplasty. This patient exhibited residual medial laxity and could be salvaged by the use of an isolated thicker modular insert exchange.

REVISION BY RESURFACING A COMPARTMENT THAT HAS UNDERGONE SECONDARY DEGENERATION

It would be tempting to salvage a UKA that has failed because of secondary degeneration of the opposite or patellofemoral compartment by retention of the UKA and adding an isolated resurfacing of that compartment. These revisions can be successful but should probably be reserved for salvaging the UKA in a younger patient. They are fraught with technical problems that can be difficult to overcome. These include providing a congruent mechanically sound patellofemoral articulation when there are now two isolated metallic femoral condylar resurfacings. If just a patellar resurfacing is added, it can be difficult to provide a smooth congruent patellofemoral articulation and transition in higher flexion angles. There are no reported long-term results in the literature utilizing secondary compartmental resurfacing in failed UKAs.

REFERENCES

1. Barrett WP, Scott RD. Revision of failed unicondylar unicompartmental knee arthroplasty. *J Bone Joint Surg Am*. 1987;69:1328–1335.
2. Levine WN, Ozuna RM, Scott RD, et al. Conversion of failed modern unicompartmental arthroplasty to total knee arthroplasty. *J Arthroplasty*. 1996;11:797–801.
3. Springer BD, Scott RD, Thornhill TS. Conversion of failed unicompartmental knee arthroplasty to TKA. *Clin Orthop*. 2006;446:214–220.
4. Lombardi Jr AV, Kolich MT, Berend KR, Morris MJ, Crawford DA, Adams JB. Revision of unicompartmental knee arthroplasty to total knee arthroplasty: is it as good as a primary result? *J Arthroplasty*. 2018;33(7S):S105–S108.
5. Lim JBT, Pang HN, Tay KJD, Chia SL, Lo NN, Yeo SJ. Clinical outcomes and patient satisfaction following revision of failed unicompartmental knee arthroplasty to total knee arthroplasty are as good as a primary total knee arthroplasty. *Knee*. 2019;26(4):847–852.
6. Schwarzkopf R, Mikhael B, Li L, Josephs L, Scott RD. Effect of initial tibial resection thickness on outcomes of revision UKA. *Orthopedics*. 2013;36(4):409–414.
7. Clark M, Campbell DG, Kiss G, Dobson PJ, Lewis PL. Reintervention after mobile-bearing Oxford unicompartmental knee arthroplasty. *Clin Orthop Relat Res*. 2010;468(2):576–580.
8. Kim KT, Lee S, Lee JI, Kim JW. Analysis and treatment of complications after unicompartmental knee arthroplasty. *Knee Surg Relat Res*. 2016;28(1):46–54.
9. Kim SG, Kim HG, Lee SY, Lim HC, Bae JH. Redislocation after bearing exchange for the treatment of mobile bearing dislocation in medial unicompartmental knee arthroplasty. *Knee Surg Relat Res*. 2018;30(3):234–240.

11

Evolving Technology in Unicompartmental Knee Arthroplasty

INTRODUCTION

The evolution of the basic technical principles of unicompartmental arthroplasty design and implantation are discussed in Chapters 1, 3, 6 and 7. These should endure for years to come. Innovative technological advances, however, will appear, evolve, and find their place in the years to come. This final chapter will discuss current evolving technologies such as robotic component positioning, patient-specific instruments and prosthetic components, and cementless fixation.

ROBOTIC COMPONENT POSITIONING

Innovative technologies have been introduced to improve component positioning with the goal of increasing the longevity of unicompartmental knee arthroplasty (UKA). Several systems have been developed including the MAKO Robotic Tactile Guidance System, the MAKO Robotic Arm Interactive Orthopedic System (MAKO RIO), Navio Precision Free-Hand Sculptor, ROBODOC, Acrobot, and UniAlign, with MAKO commanding the largest market share in robotic-assisted joint arthroplasty at the time of this publication.

Several studies have shown that robotic-assisted surgical procedures result in higher accuracy of component positioning and lower incidence of alignment outliers. In one randomized control trial, 120 patients were randomly assigned to robotic-assisted surgery or conventional UKA, and it was found that the proportion of patients within 2 degrees of the preoperative target position was significantly higher in robotic-assisted surgery for femoral component sagittal, coronal, and axial position, and tibial component sagittal and axial position.[1] In a metaanalysis of robotic-assisted versus conventional UKA, robotic-assisted UKA was similarly found to have significantly lower mechanical axis and tibial component position deviations compared with conventional UKA.[2] However, it has also been shown that an experienced, high-volume surgeon can meet or exceed robotic accuracy for tibial alignment in manual UKA.[3]

SURVIVORSHIP AND FUNCTIONAL OUTCOMES

Patients who undergo robotic-assisted UKA have high survivorship, reported as high as 98.8%, and high patient satisfaction in the short- and mid-term (2–5 years).[4,5] Whereas it is generally accepted that robotic-assistance allows for fewer component position outliers, the accuracy of component position has not necessarily translated to better survivorship or improved long-term functional outcomes. In a metaanalysis looking at pooled data from 11 studies, it showed that robotic-assisted UKA had a lower complication rate and improved knee excursion during weight acceptance.[6] Similarly, in another metaanalysis, patients who underwent robotic-assisted UKA had higher Knee Society Scores and Knee Society Function Scores at short-term follow-up (<3 years).[2] However, there was no difference in revision rates or range of motion. In the Australian National Joint Replacement Registry, they found that there was no difference in overall revision rate for robotic-assisted UKA compared to the Zimmer Unicompartmental High Flex Knee System (ZUK) in the short-term (<3 years), though there was a significantly lower revision rate for robotic-assisted UKA compared with other types of conventional UKA.[7] Similarly in a matched cohort study of a Medicare database, there was no difference in complications or revision rates at 2 years of follow-up for patients who underwent computer-assisted UKA versus standard UKA.[8] Long-term survivorship data of robotic-assisted technologies are not presently available, but long-term survivorship of UKA seems to be closely linked to surgeon caseload.[9] Thus, the benefit of better component position may be best realized with low-volume surgeons.

COST EFFECTIVENESS

Though robotic-assistance is associated with higher accuracy of component positioning, it does come at the cost of increased operative time. In a metaanalysis, it was shown that robotic-assisted surgery significantly prolonged surgical time for a mean difference of 17 minutes.[2] This may be due to the additional setup and instrumentation required for robotic-assistance or surgeon learning curve, though it has been proposed that the learning curve for the MAKO system may be as little as six cases.[10] With limited data on long-term outcomes of robotic-assisted UKA, increased cost of robotic equipment, and increased operative time, the question of cost-effectiveness arises. To address this question, one study used a Markov decision analysis model and found that robotic-assisted UKA was cost-effective compared to total knee arthroplasty (TKA) and high tibial osteotomy (HTO) under certain circumstances: (1) case volume exceeded 94 cases per year, (2) robotic-assisted UKA 2-year failure rate was below 1.2%, (3) robotic-assisted UKA provided improved failure rate beyond 2 years, (4) discounted costs of the robotic system and maintenance were less than $1.426 million, (5) the robotic system lifetime was at least 4.7 years, and (6) the average patient age was younger than 67 years.[11]

PATIENT-SPECIFIC INSTRUMENTATION AND CUSTOM IMPLANTS

Off-the-shelf UKA have a good track record, but they are not designed to restore normal knee anatomy. Theoretically, customized 3D-printed UKA implants and/or patient-specific instrumentation (PSI) (e.g., patient-specific cutting blocks) may restore normal knee anatomy and natural gait patterns with the goal of improved functional outcomes. The literature on PSI UKA is limited, where some authors have found no benefit to PSI and others have shown PSI to improve accuracy of tibial component positioning.[12–14] In a randomized control trial of 60 patients randomly assigned to UKA using PSI or by conventional technique, there was no difference in gait parameters, frontal and sagittal positioning, or Knee Society Score at 3 months and 1 year.[12] Similarly, there is limited data on the mid- to long-term outcomes of custom UKA implants, but in a prospective study of 88 patients with custom, individually-made UKA implants, the overall revision rate at 2 years was 3.3% for tibial loosening or osteoarthritis disease progression.[15] Nearly all (99%) of these patients were satisfied with their UKA, and 89% felt that movement in their knee felt natural. However, another study of 115 custom UKAs performed by one surgeon over 7 years showed that there was a 25.2% failure rate of custom UKAs at an average of 33.1 months. These failures were associated with high body mass index and were largely for aseptic loosening of the femoral component, tibial component, or both.[16] Though it is unclear what the survivorship is of custom implants, there are data to suggest that custom UKA implants outperform off-the-shelf implants in cortical bone coverage while minimizing overhang.[17] Further investigations and long-term follow-up are needed to better understand the future roles of custom implants and PSI in UKA.

CEMENTLESS FIXATION

The role of cementless fixation continues to evolve for both TKA and UKA with much less experience to date with cementless UKA. There are several reasons for this. Ideally, UKA is a conservative bone-sparing procedure. As noted in Chapter 10, minimal tibial resection is the key to allowing a UKA revision to be carried out easily without the need for modular augments to accommodate loss of tibial bone stock and the need for extended tibial stems to enhance tibial component fixation. Minimal tibial resection, however, will often create a bone bed that is more cortical in quality than cancellous, compromising bone ingrowth. A cemented tibial component allows for this ideal minimal tibial resection and the paucity of cement required for adequate component fixation will not compromise any future potential revision. Residual tibial bone defects due to cement after UKA tend to be contained, not supportive, and lend themselves to being filled with autogenous bone from the normal femoral and tibial resections needed for a TKA (see Chapter 10). Finally, cementless UKA technique is intuitively less forgiving than cemented technique and is less likely to be successful when used by less experienced surgeons.[18,19]

The published results of cementless fixation in UKA are obviously shorter term than those available for cemented components. Many reports using a mobile-bearing design do show results comparable to those obtained using cemented components.[20–23] Longer follow-up will be required, however, to prove any significant advantage of cementless over cemented UKA. More studies are also needed to assess results of cementless UKA in the hands of less experienced surgeons and with the use of fixed-bearing implants.

REFERENCES

1. Bell SW, Anthony I, Jones B, et al. Improved accuracy of component positioning with robotic-assisted unicompartmental knee arthroplasty. *J Bone Jt Surg Am*. 2016;98(8):627–635.
2. Chin BZ, Tan SSH, Chua KCX, et al. The three-year survivorship of robotically assisted versus non-robotically assisted unicompartmental knee arthroplasty. *J Arthroplasty*. 2020;33(8):1719–1926.
3. Bush AN, Ziemba-Davis M, Deckard ER, Meneghini RM. An experienced surgeon can meet or exceed robotic accuracy in manual unicompartmental knee arthroplasty. *J Bone Joint Surg Am*. 2019;101(16):1479–1484.
4. Pearle AD, van der List JP, Lee L, et al. 2017. Survivorship and patient satisfaction of robotic-assisted medial unicompartmental knee arthroplasty at a minimum two-year follow-up. Knee 24(2):419–428.
5. Flury A, Hasler J, Dimitriou D, et al. Midterm clinical and radiographic outcomes of 115 consecutive patient-specific unicompartmental knee arthroplasties. *Knee*. 2019;26(4):889–896.
6. Zhang F, Li H, Ba Z, et al. Robotic arm-assisted vs conventional unicompartmental knee arthroplasty. A meta-analysis of the effects on clinical outcomes. *Medicine*. 2019;98(35):e16968.
7. St Mart JP, De Steiger RN, Cuthbert A, Donnelly W. The three-year survivorship of robotically assisted versus non-robotically assisted unicompartmental knee arthroplasty. *Bone Joint J*. 2020;102-B(3):319–328.
8. Chona D, Bala A, Huddleston JI, et al. Effect of computer navigation on complication rates following unicompartmental knee arthroplasty. *J Arthroplasty*. 2018;33(11):3437–3440.e1.
9. Mohammad HR, Matharu GS, Judge A, Murray DW. The effect of surgeon caseload on the relative revision rate of cemented and cementless unicompartmental knee replacements: an analysis from the National Joint Registry for England, Wales, Northern Ireland and the Isle of Man. *J Bone Joint Surg Am*. 2020;102(8):644–653.
10. Kayani B, Konan S, Pietrzak JRT, et al. The learning curve associated with robotic-arm assisted unicompartmental knee arthroplasty. *Bone Joint J*. 2018;100B(8):1033–1042.
11. Moschetti WE, Konopka JF, Rubash HE, Genuario JW. Can robot-assisted unicompartmental knee arthroplasty be cost-effective? A Markov decision analysis. *J Arthroplasty*. 2016;31(4):759–765.
12. Ollivier M, Parratte S, Lunebourg A, et al. The John Insall Award: no functional benefit after unicompartmental knee arthroplasty performed with patient-specific instrumentation: a randomized trial. *Clin Orthop Relat Res*. 2016;474(1):60–68.
13. Alvand A, Khan T, Jenkins C, et al. The impact of patient-specific instrumentation on unicompartmental knee arthroplasty: a prospective randomised controlled study. *Knee Surg Sports Traumatol Arthrosc*. 2018;26(6):1662–1670.
14. Dao Trong ML, Diezi C, Goerres G, Helmy N. Improved positioning of the tibial component in unicompartmental knee arthroplasty with patient-specific cutting blocks. *Knee Surg Sports Traumatol Arthrosc*. 2015;23(7):1993–1998.
15. Sinha R, Burkhardt J, Martin G, et al. Customized, individually made unicondylar knee replacement: a prospective, multicenter study of 2-year clinical outcomes. Presented at the 2014 Harvard Arthroplasty Course.
16. Talmo CT, Anderson MC, Jia ES, et al. Primary arthroplasty high rate of early revision after custom-made unicondylar knee arthroplasty. *Primary Arthroplasty*. 2018;33(suppl 7): S100–S104.
17. Carpenter DP, Holmberg RR, Quartulli MJ, Lowry Barnes C. Tibial plateau coverage in UKA: a comparison of patient specific and off-the-shelf implants. *J Arthroplasty*. 2014;29(9):1694–1698.
18. Murray DW, Parkinson RW. Usage of unicompartmental knee arthroplasty. *Bone Joint J*. 2018;100-B(4):432–435.
19. Kamenaga T, Hiranaka T, Nakanishi Y, Takayama K, Kuroda R, Matsumoto T. Valgus subsidence of the tibial component caused by tibial component malpositioning in cementless Oxford mobile-bearing unicompartmental knee arthroplasty. *J Arthroplasty*. 2019;34(12):3054–3060.
20. Liddle AD, Pandit H, Murray DW, Dodd CA. Cementless unicondylar knee arthroplasty. *Orthop Clin North Am*. 2013;44(3):261–269.
21. Van der List JP, Sheng DL, Kleeblad LJ, Chawla H, Pearle AD. Outcomes of cementless unicompartmental and total knee arthroplasty: a systematic review. *Knee*. 2017;24(3):497–507.
22. Knifsund J, Reito A, Haapakoski J, et al. Short-term survival of cementless Oxford unicondylar knee arthroplasty based on the Finnish Arthroplasty Register. *Knee*. 2019;26(3):768–773.
23. Mohammad HR, Bullock GS, Kennedy JA, Mellon SJ, Murray D, Judge A. Cementless unicompartmental knee replacement achieves better ten-year clinical outcomes than cemented: a systematic review. *Knee Surg Sports Traumatol Arthrosc*. 2020;29(10):3229–3245.

INDEX

Page numbers followed by '*f*' indicate figures, '*t*' indicate tables.

I

K

L

M